D0730901

FREE Test Taking Tips DVD Offer

To help us better serve you, we have developed a Test Taking Tips DVD that we would like to give you for FREE. **This DVD covers world-class test taking tips that you can use to be even more successful when you are taking your test.**

All that we ask is that you email us your feedback about your study guide. Please let us know what you thought about it – whether that is good, bad or indifferent.

To get your **FREE Test Taking Tips DVD**, email freedvd@studyguideteam.com with "FREE DVD" in the subject line and the following information in the body of the email:

    a. The title of your study guide.

    b. Your product rating on a scale of 1-5, with 5 being the highest rating.

    c. Your feedback about the study guide. What did you think of it?

    d. Your full name and shipping address to send your free DVD.

If you have any questions or concerns, please don't hesitate to contact us at freedvd@studyguideteam.com.

Thanks again!

ATI TEAS Study Manual

ATI TEAS Version 6 Review Manual Team

Table of Contents

Quick Overview

As you draw closer to taking your exam, effective preparation becomes more and more important. Thankfully, you have this study guide to help you get ready. Use this guide to help keep your studying on track and refer to it often.

This study guide contains several key sections that will help you be successful on your exam. The guide contains tips for what you should do the night before and the day of the test. Also included are test-taking tips. Knowing the right information is not always enough. Many well-prepared test takers struggle with exams. These tips will help equip you to accurately read, assess, and answer test questions.

A large part of the guide is devoted to showing you what content to expect on the exam and to helping you better understand that content. Near the end of this guide is a practice test so that you can see how well you have grasped the content. Then, answer explanations are provided so that you can understand why you missed certain questions.

Don't try to cram the night before you take your exam. This is not a wise strategy for a few reasons. First, your retention of the information will be low. Your time would be better used by reviewing information you already know rather than trying to learn a lot of new information. Second, you will likely become stressed as you try to gain a large amount of knowledge in a short amount of time. Third, you will be depriving yourself of sleep. So be sure to go to bed at a reasonable time the night before. Being well-rested helps you focus and remain calm.

Be sure to eat a substantial breakfast the morning of the exam. If you are taking the exam in the afternoon, be sure to have a good lunch as well. Being hungry is distracting and can make it difficult to focus. You have hopefully spent lots of time preparing for the exam. Don't let an empty stomach get in the way of success!

When travelling to the testing center, leave earlier than needed. That way, you have a buffer in case you experience any delays. This will help you remain calm and will keep you from missing your appointment time at the testing center.

Be sure to pace yourself during the exam. Don't try to rush through the exam. There is no need to risk performing poorly on the exam just so you can leave the testing center early. Allow yourself to use all of the allotted time if needed.

Remain positive while taking the exam even if you feel like you are performing poorly. Thinking about the content you should have mastered will not help you perform better on the exam.

Once the exam is complete, take some time to relax. Even if you feel that you need to take the exam again, you will be well served by some down time before you begin studying again. It's often easier to convince yourself to study if you know that it will come with a reward!

Test-Taking Strategies

1. Predicting the Answer

When you feel confident in your preparation for a multiple-choice test, try predicting the answer before reading the answer choices. This is especially useful on questions that test objective factual knowledge or that ask you to fill in a blank. By predicting the answer before reading the available choices, you eliminate the possibility that you will be distracted or led astray by an incorrect answer choice. You will feel more confident in your selection if you read the question, predict the answer, and then find your prediction among the answer choices. After using this strategy, be sure to still read all of the answer choices carefully and completely. If you feel unprepared, you should not attempt to predict the answers. This would be a waste of time and an opportunity for your mind to wander in the wrong direction.

2. Reading the Whole Question

Too often, test takers scan a multiple-choice question, recognize a few familiar words, and immediately jump to the answer choices. Test authors are aware of this common impatience, and they will sometimes prey upon it. For instance, a test author might subtly turn the question into a negative, or he or she might redirect the focus of the question right at the end. The only way to avoid falling into these traps is to read the entirety of the question carefully before reading the answer choices.

3. Looking for Wrong Answers

Long and complicated multiple-choice questions can be intimidating. One way to simplify a difficult multiple-choice question is to eliminate all of the answer choices that are clearly wrong. In most sets of answers, there will be at least one selection that can be dismissed right away. If the test is administered on paper, the test taker could draw a line through it to indicate that it may be ignored; otherwise, the test taker will have to perform this operation mentally or on scratch paper. In either case, once the obviously incorrect answers have been eliminated, the remaining choices may be considered. Sometimes identifying the clearly wrong answers will give the test taker some information about the correct answer. For instance, if one of the remaining answer choices is a direct opposite of one of the eliminated answer choices, it may well be the correct answer. The opposite of obviously wrong is obviously right! Of course, this is not always the case. Some answers are obviously incorrect simply because they are irrelevant to the question being asked. Still, identifying and eliminating some incorrect answer choices is a good way to simplify a multiple-choice question.

4. Don't Overanalyze

Anxious test takers often overanalyze questions. When you are nervous, your brain will often run wild, causing you to make associations and discover clues that don't actually exist. If you feel that this may be a problem for you, do whatever you can to slow down during the test. Try taking a deep breath or counting to ten. As you read and consider the question, restrict yourself to the particular words used by the author. Avoid thought tangents about what the author *really* meant, or what he or she was *trying* to say. The only things that matter on a multiple-choice test are the words that are actually in the question. You must avoid reading too much into a multiple-choice question, or supposing that the writer meant something other than what he or she wrote.

5. No Need for Panic

It is wise to learn as many strategies as possible before taking a multiple-choice test, but it is likely that you will come across a few questions for which you simply don't know the answer. In this situation, avoid panicking. Because most multiple-choice tests include dozens of questions, the relative value of a single wrong answer is small. Moreover, your failure on one question has no effect on your success elsewhere on the test. As much as possible, you should compartmentalize each question on a multiple-choice test. In other words, you should not allow your feelings about one question to affect your success on the others. When you find a question that you either don't understand or don't know how to answer, just take a deep breath and do your best. Read the entire question slowly and carefully. Try rephrasing the question a couple of different ways. Then, read all of the answer choices carefully. After eliminating obviously wrong answers, make a selection and move on to the next question.

6. Confusing Answer Choices

When working on a difficult multiple-choice question, there may be a tendency to focus on the answer choices that are the easiest to understand. Many people, whether consciously or not, gravitate to the answer choices that require the least concentration, knowledge, and memory. This is a mistake. When you come across an answer choice that is confusing, you should give it extra attention. A question might be confusing because you do not know the subject matter to which it refers. If this is the case, don't eliminate the answer before you have affirmatively settled on another. When you come across an answer choice of this type, set it aside as you look at the remaining choices. If you can confidently assert that one of the other choices is correct, you can leave the confusing answer aside. Otherwise, you will need to take a moment to try to better understand the confusing answer choice. Rephrasing is one way to tease out the sense of a confusing answer choice.

7. Your First Instinct

Many people struggle with multiple-choice tests because they overthink the questions. If you have studied sufficiently for the test, you should be prepared to trust your first instinct once you have carefully and completely read the question and all of the answer choices. There is a great deal of research suggesting that the mind can come to the correct conclusion very quickly once it has obtained all of the relevant information. At times, it may seem to you as if your intuition is working faster even than your reasoning mind. This may in fact be true. The knowledge you obtain while studying may be retrieved from your subconscious before you have a chance to work out the associations that support it. Verify your instinct by working out the reasons that it should be trusted.

8. Key Words

Many test takers struggle with multiple-choice questions because they have poor reading comprehension skills. Quickly reading and understanding a multiple-choice question requires a mixture of skill and experience. To help with this, try jotting down a few key words and phrases on a piece of scrap paper. Doing this concentrates the process of reading and forces the mind to weigh the relative importance of the question's parts. In selecting words and phrases to write down, the test taker thinks about the question more deeply and carefully. This is especially true for multiple-choice questions that are preceded by a long prompt.

9. Subtle Negatives

One of the oldest tricks in the multiple-choice test writer's book is to subtly reverse the meaning of a question with a word like *not* or *except*. If you are not paying attention to each word in the question, you can easily be led astray by this trick. For instance, a common question format is, "Which of the following is…?" Obviously, if the question instead is, "Which of the following is not…?," then the answer will be quite different. Even worse, the test makers are aware of the potential for this mistake and will include one answer choice that would be correct if the question were not negated or reversed. A test taker who misses the reversal will find what he or she believes to be a correct answer and will be so confident that he or she will fail to reread the question and discover the original error. The only way to avoid this is to practice a wide variety of multiple-choice questions and to pay close attention to each and every word.

10. Reading Every Answer Choice

It may seem obvious, but you should always read every one of the answer choices! Too many test takers fall into the habit of scanning the question and assuming that they understand the question because they recognize a few key words. From there, they pick the first answer choice that answers the question they believe they have read. Test takers who read all of the answer choices might discover that one of the latter answer choices is actually *more* correct. Moreover, reading all of the answer choices can remind you of facts related to the question that can help you arrive at the correct answer. Sometimes, a misstatement or incorrect detail in one of the latter answer choices will trigger your memory of the subject and will enable you to find the right answer. Failing to read all of the answer choices is like not reading all of the items on a restaurant menu: you might miss out on the perfect choice.

11. Spot the Hedges

One of the keys to success on multiple-choice tests is paying close attention to every word. This is never more true than with words like *almost*, *most*, *some*, and *sometimes*. These words are called "hedges" because they indicate that a statement is not totally true or not true in every place and time. An absolute statement will contain no hedges, but in many subjects, like literature and history, the answers are not always straightforward or absolute. There are always exceptions to the rules in these subjects. For this reason, you should favor those multiple-choice questions that contain hedging language. The presence of qualifying words indicates that the author is taking special care with his or her words, which is certainly important when composing the right answer. After all, there are many ways to be wrong, but there is only one way to be right! For this reason, it is wise to avoid answers that are absolute when taking a multiple-choice test. An absolute answer is one that says things are either all one way or all another. They often include words like *every*, *always*, *best*, and *never*. If you are taking a multiple-choice test in a subject that doesn't lend itself to absolute answers, be on your guard if you see any of these words.

12. Long Answers

In many subject areas, the answers are not simple. As already mentioned, the right answer often requires hedges. Another common feature of the answers to a complex or subjective question are qualifying clauses, which are groups of words that subtly modify the meaning of the sentence. If the question or answer choice describes a rule to which there are exceptions or the subject matter is complicated, ambiguous, or confusing, the correct answer will require many words in order to be expressed clearly and accurately. In essence, you should not be deterred by answer choices that seem excessively long. Oftentimes, the author of the text will not be able to write the correct answer without offering some qualifications and modifications. Your job is to read the answer choices thoroughly and completely and to select the one that most accurately and precisely answers the question.

13. Restating to Understand

Sometimes, a question on a multiple-choice test is difficult not because of what it asks but because of how it is written. If this is the case, restate the question or answer choice in different words. This process serves a couple of important purposes. First, it forces you to concentrate on the core of the question. In order to rephrase the question accurately, you have to understand it well. Rephrasing the question will concentrate your mind on the key words and ideas. Second, it will present the information to your mind in a fresh way. This process may trigger your memory and render some useful scrap of information picked up while studying.

14. True Statements

Sometimes an answer choice will be true in itself, but it does not answer the question. This is one of the main reasons why it is essential to read the question carefully and completely before proceeding to the answer choices. Too often, test takers skip ahead to the answer choices and look for true statements. Having found one of these, they are content to select it without reference to the question above. Obviously, this provides an easy way for test makers to play tricks. The savvy test taker will always read the entire question before turning to the answer choices. Then, having settled on a correct answer choice, he or she will refer to the original question and ensure that the selected answer is relevant. The mistake of choosing a correct-but-irrelevant answer choice is especially common on questions related to specific pieces of objective knowledge, like historical or scientific facts. A prepared test taker will have a wealth of factual knowledge at his or her disposal, and should not be careless in its application.

15. No Patterns

One of the more dangerous ideas that circulates about multiple-choice tests is that the correct answers tend to fall into patterns. These erroneous ideas range from a belief that B and C are the most common right answers, to the idea that an unprepared test-taker should answer "A-B-A-C-A-D-A-B-A." It cannot be emphasized enough that pattern-seeking of this type is exactly the WRONG way to approach a multiple-choice test. To begin with, it is highly unlikely that the test maker will plot the correct answers according to some predetermined pattern. The questions are scrambled and delivered in a random order. Furthermore, even if the test maker was following a pattern in the assignation of correct answers, there is no reason why the test taker would know which pattern he or she was using. Any attempt to discern a pattern in the answer choices is a waste of time and a distraction from the real work of taking the test. A test taker would be much better served by extra preparation before the test than by reliance on a pattern in the answers.

FREE DVD OFFER

Don't forget that doing well on your exam includes both understanding the test content and understanding how to use what you know to do well on the test. We offer a completely FREE Test Taking Tips DVD that covers world class test taking tips that you can use to be even more successful when you are taking your test.

All that we ask is that you email us your feedback about your study guide. To get your **FREE Test Taking Tips DVD**, email freedvd@studyguideteam.com with "FREE DVD" in the subject line and the following information in the body of the email:

- The title of your study guide.
- Your product rating on a scale of 1-5, with 5 being the highest rating.
- Your feedback about the study guide. What did you think of it?
- Your full name and shipping address to send your free DVD.

Introduction the ATI TEAS

Background of the ATI TEAS

The Test of Essential Academic Skills (TEAS) is a standardized test created and distributed by Assessment Technologies Institute (ATI) to examine the test taker's aptitude for skill sets fundamental to a career in nursing. As such, the TEAS is used by nursing schools and allied health schools in the United States and Canada as a chief criterion for admission. The TEAS is currently in its sixth iteration, known as the ATI TEAS.

The ATI TEAS is a nationwide test, with no variation in the difficulty of content among the versions given from state to state; the content of the TEAS is a standard measure for entry-level skills and abilities for nursing applicants. However, the required minimum TEAS scores, like prerequisite courses or application distinctions, can vary widely between schools and programs. Because the TEAS is used for admission to nursing and allied health programs, the majority of TEAS takers are high school diploma or GED graduates pursuing a career in nursing or are applicants to programs requiring prerequisite academic coursework. These applicants can range in background from sophomore-level collegiate to professionals looking to change careers into a healthcare field.

Test Administration

The ATI TEAS may be administered by a nursing or allied health school or a PSI testing center. The testing schedule is chosen by each individual facility, and the regularity of testing can vary from major metropolitan areas (where it may be offered multiple times per week in several locations) to sparsely populated towns (where it may be offered once per month every hundred miles). The test will also be proctored to make certain that testing protocols are enforced. Test takers can register at atitesting.com or directly through the school to which they wish to apply, as most nursing schools offer the test on-campus periodically throughout the year. The cost to take the ATI TEAS is set by the local administrator, but it usually ranges from $83 to $105.

Students may retake the ATI TEAS, but most schools have limitations such as the number of days students must wait between attempts, or the number of attempts students may make in a given period. For instance, many schools will accept the higher score of two attempts within a twelve-month period, but will not consider a third attempt until twelve months has lapsed since the first attempt. Disability accommodations are generally available and made by contacting the local test administration site.

Test Format

The ATI TEAS is comprised of 170 multiple choice questions with four possible answer choices given for each question. The questions are divided between four subject areas—Reading, Mathematics, Science, and English and Language Usage.

Subject Area	Questions	Time Limit
Reading	53	64
Mathematics	36	54
Science	53	63
English & Language Usage	28	28
Total	**170**	**209**

Test takers are given 209 minutes to take the ATI TEAS, broken down among the four subject areas. Once a test taker begins a subject area, the timer will start. When the timer expires, the test taker may stretch, go to the bathroom, or otherwise relax before the timer begins for the next section. The ATI TEAS is offered in both a pencil-and-paper version and a computerized version, depending on the preference of the local test administrator. ATI TEAS test takers are not permitted to use cell phones, but four-function calculators are permitted now on the ATI TEAS.

Scoring

Shortly after the examination, test takers will receive several different numbered scores with their ATI TEAS results, including scores on all the various sections and subsections. This includes the national and state-level percentile rankings that a test taker has achieved. This rank is equal to the percentage of test takers from nationwide samples that scored equal to or lower than the test taker. Higher percentiles indicate more correct answers and fewer people who scored higher than the given test taker. However, although this may be of interest to the test taker, schools do not use this score to base acceptance decisions on.

Instead, schools typically look at the Composite Individual Total Score. The composite score is a good determination of the performance of the test taker and is calculated by averaging the test taker's performance from each section of the test. The national average composite score generally lies between 65% correct and 75% correct, and many schools have a minimum required score in this range, but each school and program chooses their own minimum standards; more prestigious schools require higher minimum scores and vice versa. Besides meeting minimum requirements, TEAS scores can play a part in the acceptance process as one of the factors like previous GPAs and extracurricular activities that demonstrate the competitiveness of the applicant, but this too varies from school to school.

Recent Developments

ATI TEAS is the sixth version of the TEAS, and is offered starting August 31, 2016. Before August 31, 2016, the fifth version of the TEAS (known as the TEAS V) was the current version of the TEAS. The ATI TEAS is similar in difficulty, but with slight differences in the amount of emphasis placed on various subjects, such as the reduction of the English & Language Usage section and the elimination of the Earth Science subsection. Four-function calculators are now permitted on the ATI TEAS.

Reading

Key Ideas and Details

Summarizing a Complex Text

A summary is a shortened version of the original text, written by the reader in their own words. In order to effectively summarize a more complex text, it is necessary to fully understand the original source, and to highlight the major points covered. It may be helpful to outline the original text to get a big picture view of it, and to avoid getting bogged down in the minor details. For example, a summary wouldn't need to include a specific statistic from the original source unless it was the major focus of the piece. Also, it's important for readers to use their own words, but to retain the original meaning of the passage. The key to a good summary is to emphasize the main idea without changing the focus of the original information.

Paraphrasing calls for the reader to take a small part of the passage and list or describe its main points. Paraphrasing is more than rewording the original passage, though. Like summary, it should be written in the reader's own words, while still retaining the meaning of the original source. The main difference between summarizing and paraphrasing is the length of the original passage. A summary would be appropriate for a much larger piece, while paraphrase might focus on just a few lines of text. Effective paraphrasing will indicate an understanding of the original source, yet still help the reader expand on their interpretation. A paraphrase should neither add new information nor remove essential facts that will change the meaning of the source.

Inferring the Logical Conclusion from a Reading Selection

Determining conclusions requires being an active reader, as a reader must make a prediction and analyze facts to identify a conclusion. A reader should identify key words in a passage to determine the logical conclusion or determination that flows from the information presented. Consider the passage below:

Lindsay, covered in flour, moved around the kitchen frantically. Her mom yelled from another room, "Lindsay, we're going to be late!

You can conclude that Lindsay's next steps are to finish baking, clean herself up, and head off somewhere with her baked goods. Notice that the conclusion cannot be verified factually. Many conclusions are not spelled out specifically in the text, thus they have to be identified and drawn out by the reader.

Identifying the Topic, Main Idea, and Supporting Details

Topic Versus the Main Idea
It is very important to know the difference between the topic and the main idea of the text. Even though these two are similar because they both present the central point of a text, they have distinctive differences. A *topic* is the subject of the text; it can usually be described in a one- to two-word phrase and appears in the simplest form. On the other hand, the *main idea* is more detailed and provides the author's central point of the text. It can be expressed through a complete sentence and is often found in the beginning, middle, or end of a paragraph. In most nonfiction books, the first sentence of the passage usually (but not always) states the main idea

Review the passage below to explore the topic versus the main idea:

Cheetahs

Cheetahs are one of the fastest mammals on the land, reaching up to 70 miles an hour over short distances. Even though cheetahs can run as fast as 70 miles an hour, they usually only have to run half that speed to catch up with their choice of prey. Cheetahs cannot maintain a fast pace over long periods of time because their bodies will overheat. After a chase, cheetahs need to rest for approximately 30 minutes prior to eating or returning to any other activity.

In the example above, the topic of the passage is "Cheetahs" simply because that is the subject of the text. The main idea of the text is "Cheetahs are one of the fastest mammals on the land but can only maintain a fast pace for shorter distances." While it covers the topic, it is more detailed and refers to the text in its entirety. The text continues to provide additional details called *supporting details,* which will be discussed in the next section.

Supporting Details

Supporting details help readers better develop and understand the main idea. Supporting details answer questions like *who, what, where, when, why,* and *how.* Different types of supporting details include examples, facts and statistics, anecdotes, and sensory details.

Persuasive and informative texts often use supporting details. In persuasive texts, authors attempt to make readers agree with their points of view, and supporting details are often used as "selling points." If authors make a statement, they need to support the statement with evidence in order to adequately persuade readers. Informative texts use supporting details such as examples and facts to inform readers. Review the previous "Cheetahs" passage to find examples of supporting details.

Cheetahs

Cheetahs are one of the fastest mammals on the land, reaching up to 70 miles an hour over short distances. Even though cheetahs can run as fast as 70 miles an hour, they usually only have to run half that speed to catch up with their choice of prey. Cheetahs cannot maintain a fast pace over long periods of time because their bodies will overheat. After a chase, cheetahs need to rest for approximately 30 minutes prior to eating or returning to any other activity.

In the example, supporting details include:

- Cheetahs reach up to 70 miles per hour over short distances.
- They usually only have to run half that speed to catch up with their prey.
- Cheetahs will overheat if they exert a high speed over longer distances.
- Cheetahs need to rest for 30 minutes after a chase.

Look at the diagram below (applying the cheetah example) to help determine the hierarchy of topic, main idea, and supporting details.

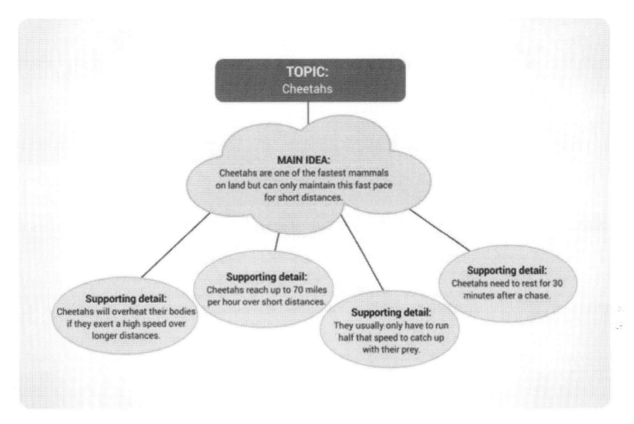

Following a Given Set of Directions

When you read a comic or magazine, it's not necessary to understand everything. However, other more technical readings, such as directions for setting up a coffeemaker or a new phone app, require more attention to detail. Read each step all the way through, and don't skip ahead. While you may think that you know all or some of the steps, it's important to read directions in the manner that the writer intended. This aids in comprehension and ensures that you catch all relevant information. Take your time and reread sentences and passages if necessary. Look up unfamiliar words or concepts, and jot comments, called annotations, in the margins.

Identifying Specific Information from a Printed Communication

While expository in nature, memorandums (memos) are designed to convey basic information in a specific and concise message. Memos have a heading, which includes the information *to, from, date,* and *subject,* and a body, which is either in paragraph form or bullet points that detail what was in the subject line.

Though e-mails often replace memos in the modern workplace, printed memos still have a place. For example, if a supervisor wants to relate information, such as a company-wide policy change, to a large group, posting a memo in a staff lounge or other heavily traveled area is an efficient way to do so.

Posted announcements are useful to convey information to a large group of people. Announcements, however, take on a more informal tone than a memo. Common announcement topics include items for sale, services offered, lost pets, or business openings. Since posted announcements are found in public places, like grocery or hardware stores, they include contact information, purpose, meeting times, and prices, as well as pictures, graphics, and colors to attract the reader's eye.

Classified advertisements are another useful medium to convey information to large groups. Consider using classified advertisements when you want to buy and sell items, or look for services. Classified ads are found in newspapers, or online through *Craigslist*, *eBay*, or similar websites and blogs. While newspapers rely on ads to help fund their publications and often provide only local exposure, online sites provide a statewide or even global platform, thus shipping costs are an important consideration when looking at the cost of the item.

Regardless of the medium, all advertisements offer basic information, such as the item in question, a description, picture, cost, and the seller's contact information. It may also note a willingness to negotiate on the price or offer an option to trade in lieu of a sale. As websites like *Craigslist* and *Buy/Sell/Trade* increase in popularity, more localities offer "safe zones," where purchases and trades are conducted in supervised environments.

Identifying Information from a Graphic Representation of Information

Texts may have graphic representations to help illustrate and visually support assertions made. For example, graphics can be used to express samples or segments of a population or demonstrate growth or decay. Three of the most popular graphic formats include line graphs, bar graphs, and pie charts.

Line graphs rely on a horizontal X axis and a vertical Y axis to establish baseline values. Dots are plotted where the horizontal and vertical axes intersect, and those dots are connected with lines. Compared to bar graphs or pie charts, line graphs are more useful for looking at the past and present and predicting future outcomes. For instance, a potential investor would look for stocks that demonstrated steady growth over many decades when examining the stock market. Note that severe spikes up and down indicate instability, while line graphs that display a slow but steady increase may indicate good returns.

Here's an example of a bar graph:

Bar graphs are usually displayed on a vertical Y axis. The bars themselves can be two- or three-dimensional, depending on the designer's tastes. Unlike a line graph, which shows the fluctuation of only one variable, the X axis on a bar graph is excellent for making comparisons, because it shows differences between several variables. For instance, if a consumer wanted to buy a new tablet, she could narrow the selection down to a few choices by using a bar graph to plot the prices side by side. The tallest bar would be the most expensive tablet, the shortest bar would be the cheapest.

A pie chart is divided into wedges that represent a numerical piece of the whole. Pie charts are useful for demonstrating how different categories add up to 100 percent. However, pie charts are not useful in comparing dissimilar items. High schools tend to use pie charts to track where students end up after graduation. Each wedge, for instance, might be labeled *vocational school*, *two-year college*, *four-year college*, *workforce*, or *unemployed*. By calculating the size of each wedge, schools can offer classes in the same ratios as where students will end up after high school. Pie charts are also useful for tracking finances. Items like car payments, insurance, rent, credit cards, and entertainment would each get their own wedge proportional to the amount spent in a given time period. If one wedge is inordinately bigger than the rest, or if a wedge is expendable, it might be time to create a new financial strategy.

Identifying Scale Readings

Most measuring instruments have scales to allow someone to determine precise measurement. Many of these instruments are becoming digitized such that the screens output measurement; for example, weighing scales and tire-pressure gauges often have digital screens. However, it's still important to know how to read scales. Many rulers have scales for inches on one side and scales for centimeters on the other side. On the inches' side, the longest black lines indicate the inch marks, and the slightly shorter lines indicate the half-inch marks. Progressively shorter black lines indicate the quarter-inch, eighth-inch, and sometimes even sixteenth-inch marks.

Using Legends and Map Keys

Legends and map keys are placed on maps to identify what the symbols on the map represent. Generally map symbols stand for things like railroads, national or state highways, and public parks. Legends and maps keys can generally be found in the bottom right corner of a map. They are necessary to avoid the needless repetition of the same information because of the large amounts of information condensed onto a map. In addition there may be a compass rose that shows the directions of north, south, east, and west. Most maps are oriented such that the top of the map is north.

Maps also have scales, which are a type of legend or key that show relative distances between fixed points. If you were on a highway and nearly out of gas, a map's scale would help you determine if you could make it to the next town before running out of fuel.

Evaluating Product Information to Determine the most Economical Buy

When evaluating product information, be on the lookout for bolded and italicized words and numbers, which indicate the information is especially important. Also be on the lookout for repeated or similar information, which indicates importance. If you're trying to find the best deal, it might be useful to do a side-by-side comparison. Using software, like Microsoft Excel, can help you organize and compare costs systematically.

In addition, being a savvy shopper in today's market means not only having a decent grasp of math, but also understanding how retailers use established techniques to encourage consumers to spend more. Look for units of measurement—pounds, ounces, liters, grams, etc.—then divide the amount by the cost. By comparing this way, you may find products on sale cost more than ones that are not.

You should also take into consideration any tax or shipping costs. Obviously, the more an item costs, the more tax or shipping tends to cost too. Most brick and mortar establishments, like Target, Walmart, and Sears, are required to charge tax based on location, but some internet sites, like Amazon, Overstock, and eBay, will offer no tax or free shipping as an incentive. Comparisons between local stores and internet sites can aid in finding the best deal.

Recognizing Events in a Sequence

Sequence structure (sometimes referred to as the order structure) is when the order of events proceed in a predictable order. In many cases, this means the text goes through the plot elements: exposition, rising action, climax, falling action, and resolution. Readers are introduced to characters, setting, and conflict in the exposition. In the rising action, there's an increase in tension and suspense. The climax is the height of tension and the point of no return. Tension decreases during the falling action. In the resolution, any conflicts presented in the exposition are solved, and the story concludes.

Here's a common sequence:

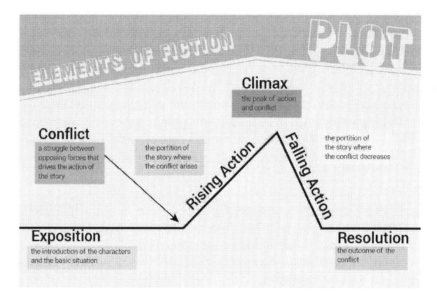

An informative text that is structured sequentially will often go in order from one step to the next.

Craft and Structure

Distinguishing Between Fact and Opinion, Biases, and Stereotypes

A fact is information that can be proven true. If information can be disproved, it is not a fact. For example, water freezes at or below thirty-two degrees Fahrenheit. An argument stating that water freezes at seventy degrees Fahrenheit cannot be supported by data, and is therefore not a fact. Facts tend to be associated with science, mathematics, and statistics.

Opinions are information open to debate. Opinions are often tied to subjective concepts like equality, morals, and rights. They can also be controversial. An affirmative argument for a position—such as gun control—can be just as effective as an opposing argument against it.

Biases and stereotypes are viewpoints based in opinion and held despite evidence that they are incorrect. A bias is an individual prejudice. Biased people ignore evidence that contradicts their position while offering as proof any evidence that supports it. A stereotype is a widely held belief projected onto a group. Those who stereotype tend to make assumptions based on what others have told them and usually have little firsthand experience with the group or item in question.

Readers must read critically to discern between fact and opinion and to notice bias and stereotypes.

Recognizing the Structure of Texts in Various Formats

Writing can be classified under four passage types: narrative, expository, technical, and persuasive. Though these types are not mutually exclusive, one form tends to dominate the rest. By recognizing the *type* of passage you're reading, you gain insight into *how* you should read. If you're reading a narrative, you can assume the author intends to entertain, which means you may skim the text without losing meaning. A technical document might require a close read, because skimming the passage might cause the reader to miss salient details.

1. *Narrative* writing, at its core, is the art of storytelling. For a narrative to exist, certain elements must be present. It must have characters. While many characters are human, characters could be defined as anything that thinks, acts, and talks like a human. For example, many recent movies, such as *Lord of the Rings* and *The Chronicles of Narnia*, include animals, fantastical creatures, and even trees that behave like humans. It must have a plot or sequence of events. Typically, those events follow a standard plot diagram, but recent trends start *in medias res* or in the middle (near the climax). In this instance, foreshadowing and flashbacks often fill in plot details. Along with characters and a plot, there must also be conflict. Conflict is usually divided into two types: internal and external. Internal conflict indicates the character is in turmoil. Internal conflicts are presented through the character's thoughts. External conflicts are visible. Types of external conflict include a person versus nature, another person, and society.

2. *Expository* writing is detached and to the point, while other types of writing—persuasive, narrative, and descriptive—are lively. Since expository writing is designed to instruct or inform, it usually involves directions and steps written in second person ("you" voice) and lacks any persuasive or narrative elements. Sequence words such as *first*, *second*, and *third*, or *in the first place*, *secondly*, and *lastly* are often given to add fluency and cohesion. Common examples of expository writing include instructor's lessons, cookbook recipes, and repair manuals.

3. Due to its empirical nature, *technical* writing is filled with steps, charts, graphs, data, and statistics. The goal of technical writing is to advance understanding in a field through the scientific method. Experts such as teachers, doctors, or mechanics use words unique to the profession in which they operate. These words, which often incorporate acronyms, are called *jargon*. Technical writing is a type of expository writing, but is not meant to be understood by the general public. Instead, technical writers assume readers have received a formal education in a particular field of study, and need no explanation as to what the jargon means. Imagine a doctor trying to understand a diagnostic reading for a car or a mechanic trying to interpret lab results. Only professionals with proper training will fully comprehend the text.

4. *Persuasive* writing is designed to change opinions and attitudes. The topic, stance, and arguments are found in the thesis, positioned near the end of the introduction. Later supporting paragraphs offer relevant quotations, paraphrases, and summaries from primary or secondary sources, which are then interpreted, analyzed, and evaluated. The goal of persuasive writers is not to stack quotes, but to develop original ideas by using sources as a starting point. Good persuasive writing makes powerful arguments with valid sources and thoughtful analysis. Poor persuasive writing is riddled with bias and logical fallacies. Sometimes, logical and illogical arguments are sandwiched together in the same piece. Therefore, readers should display skepticism when reading persuasive arguments.

Interpreting the Meaning of Words and Phrases Using Context

Most experts agree that learning new words is worth your time. It helps you understand what you're reading, and it expands your vocabulary. An extensive vocabulary improves your ability to think. When you add words to your vocabulary, you are better able to make sense of the world around you.

One of the fastest ways to decode a word is through context. Context, or surrounding words, gives clues as to what unknown words mean. Take the following example: *When the students in the classroom teased Johnny, he was so discombobulated that he couldn't finish a simple math problem.* Even though you might be unfamiliar with the word *discombobulated*, you can use context clues in the sentence to make sense of the word. In this case, you can deduce that *discombobulated* means confused or distracted.

Determining the Denotative Meaning of Words

Connotation refers to the implied meaning of a word or phrase. Connotations are the ideas or feelings that words or phrase invoke other than their literal meaning. An example of the use of connotation is in people's use of the word *cheap*. While the literal meaning is something of low cost, people use the word to suggest something is poor in value or to negatively describe a person as reluctant to spend money. When something or someone is described this way, the reader is more inclined to have a particular image or feeling about it or him/her. Thus, connotation can be a very effective language tool in creating emotion and swaying opinion. However, connotations are sometimes hard to pin down because varying emotions can be associated with a word. Generally, though, connotative meanings tend to be fairly consistent within a specific cultural group.

Denotation is the literal definition of a word or phrase. The denotative meaning of a word is the one you would find in a dictionary. To present hard facts or vocabulary terms, it is helpful for a writer to use words which are mainly known for their denotative meanings rather than their connotative ones. In those instances, the words *inexpensive* and *frugal* are better because they do not carry the negative connotations that cheap does. *Inexpensive* refers to the cost of something, not its value, and *frugal* indicates that a person is conscientiously watching his or her spending. These terms do not elicit the same emotions that *cheap* does.

Authors sometimes choose to use both, but what they choose and when they use it is what critical readers need to differentiate. One method isn't inherently better than the other; however, one may create a better effect, depending upon an author's intent. If, for example, an author's purpose is to inform, to instruct, and to familiarize readers with a difficult subject, his or her use of connotation may be helpful. However, it may also undermine credibility and confuse readers. An author who wants to create a credible, scholarly effect in his or her text would most likely use denotation, which emphasizes literal, factual meaning and examples.

Use a dictionary to find the denotative meaning of words. Though context clues provide a rudimentary understanding of a word, using a dictionary can provide the reader with a more comprehensive meaning of the word. Printed dictionaries list words in alphabetical order, and all versions, including those online, include a word's multiples meanings. Typically, the first definition is the most widely used or known. The second, third, and subsequent entries move toward the more unusual or archaic. Dictionaries also indicate the part of speech of each word, such as noun, verb, adjective, etc.

Keep in mind that dictionaries are not fixed in time. The English language today looks nothing like it did in Shakespeare's time, and Shakespeare's English is vastly different from Chaucer's. The English language is constantly evolving, as evidenced by the deletion of old words and the addition of new. *Ginormous* and *bling-bling*, for example, can both be found in *Merriam-Webster's* latest edition.

Evaluating the Author's Purpose in a Given Text

No matter the genre or format, all authors are writing to persuade, inform, entertain, or express feelings. Often, these purposes are blended, with one dominating the rest. It's useful to learn to recognize the author's intent.

Persuasive writing is used to persuade or convince readers of something. It often contains two elements: the argument and the counterargument. The argument takes a stance on an issue, while the counterargument pokes holes in the opposition's stance. Authors rely on logic, emotion, and writer credibility to persuade readers to agree with them. If readers are opposed to the stance before reading, they are unlikely to adopt that stance. However, those who are undecided or committed to the same stance are more likely to agree with the author.

Informative writing tries to teach or inform. Workplace manuals, instructor lessons, statistical reports and cookbooks are examples of informative texts. Informative writing is usually based on facts and is often void of emotion and persuasion. Informative texts generally contain statistics, charts, and graphs. Though most informative texts lack a persuasive agenda, readers must examine the text carefully to determine whether one exists within a given passage.

Stories or narratives are designed to entertain. When you go to the movies, you often want to escape for a few hours, not necessarily to think critically. Entertaining writing is designed to delight and engage the reader. However, sometimes this type of writing can be woven into more serious materials, such as persuasive or informative writing to hook the reader before transitioning into a more scholarly discussion.

Emotional writing works to evoke the reader's feelings, such as anger, euphoria, or sadness. The connection between reader and author is an attempt to cause the reader to share the author's intended emotion or tone. Sometimes in order to make a piece more poignant, the author simply wants readers to feel emotion that the author has felt. Other times, the author attempts to persuade or manipulate the reader into adopting his stance. While it's okay to sympathize with the author, be aware of the individual's underlying intent.

Evaluating the Author's Point of View in a Given Text

When it comes to authors' writings, readers should always identify a position or stance. No matter how objective a piece may seem, assume the author has preconceived beliefs. Reduce the likelihood of accepting an invalid argument by looking for multiple articles on the topic, including those with varying opinions. If several opinions point in the same direction, and are backed by reputable peer-reviewed sources, it's more likely the author has a valid argument. Positions that run contrary to widely held beliefs and existing data should invite scrutiny. There are exceptions to the rule, so be a careful consumer of information.

Though themes, symbols, and motifs are buried deep within the text and can sometimes be difficult to infer, an author's purpose is usually obvious from the beginning. There are four purposes of writing: to inform, to persuade, to describe, and to entertain. Informative writings present facts in an accessible way. Persuasive writing is appeals to emotions and logic to inspire the reader to adopt a specific stance. Be wary of this type of writing, as it often lacks objectivity. Descriptive writing is designed to paint a picture in the reader's mind, while writings that entertain are often narratives designed to engage and delight the reader.

The various writing styles are usually blended, with one purpose dominating the rest. For example, a persuasive piece might begin with a humorous tale to make readers more receptive to the persuasive message, or a recipe in a cookbook designed to inform might be preceded by an entertaining anecdote that makes the recipe more appealing.

Using Text Features

Text features are used to bring clarity or to affect the meaning of it. Sometimes a publication will follow a certain style guide/manual of style, which is a set of standards for how to write and format a publication. Some examples are APA, MLA, and the Chicago Manual of Style. If the publication is following one of those standards then the text features will be in accordance with that style guide.

Writers can come up with their own uses for text features based on what they feel is best. However, text features are generally used for a specific purpose. It's important to catch on to that purpose to maximize comprehension.

A clear layout is essential for good reader comprehension. Even with the use of many text features, the text needs to be laid out in a clear, consistent manner.

Bolding, Italics, and Underlining
Bolding, italics, and underlining are all used to make words stand out. **Bolded** words are often key concepts and can usually be found in summary statements at the end of chapters and in indexes. *Italics* can be used to identify words of another language or to add extra emphasis to a word or phrase. Writers will sometime place words in italics when the word is being referred to as the word itself. Quotation marks or italics can be used for this, as long as there is consistency. Italics are also used to represent a character's thoughts.

> Entering Jessica's room, Jessica's mom stepped over a pile of laundry, a stack of magazines, and a pile of dishes. *My messy daughter*, she thought, shaking her head.

Text can be <u>underlined</u> for a number of reasons, but generally it's to indicate a key term or important point.

Color can also be a text feature, as different color text can be used to make certain parts stand out or to indicate that a new section is beginning. Even if something is in black & white, the text may be in different shades of grey.

Formatting
In addition, formatting—such as indentation or bullet points—helps to clearly present content. Content may also be left justified, centered, or right justified:

Left Justified

Centered

Right Justified

Text is often centered to stand out and catch the reader's eye.

Using Legends and Map Keys
Legends and map keys are placed on maps to identify what the symbols on the map represent. Generally map symbols stand for things like railroads, national or state highways, and public parks. Legends and maps keys can generally be found in the bottom right corner of a map. They are necessary to avoid the needless repetition of the same information because of the large amounts of information condensed onto a map. In addition there may be a compass rose that shows the directions of north, south, east, and west. Most maps are oriented such that the top of the map is north.

Maps also have scales, which are a type of legend or key that show relative distances between fixed points. If you were on a highway and nearly out of gas, a map's scale would help you determine if you could make it to the next town before running out of fuel.

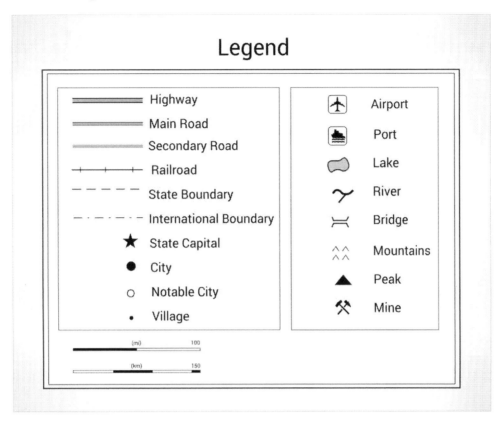

Analyzing Headings and Subheadings

Headings and subheadings are used in writing to organize discussions and allow the reader to find information quickly. Headings show a complete change in thought. Subheadings, which fall below headings, show different aspects of the same topic. For instance, if you saw the title *Government* and the heading *Forms of Government*, you might see the subheadings *Monarchy*, *Oligarchy*, *Democracy*, *Socialism*, and *Totalitarianism*.

Note the headings that got you to this point:

Reading

Key Ideas and Details

Using Text Features

As well as providing organization and structure, headings and subheadings also put more white space on a page, which places less strain on the reader's eyes. It's a good idea to skim a document and get familiar with headings and subheadings. Write down the title, headings, and subheadings before you begin reading to provide structure to your notes and thoughts.

<u>Identifying Information from a Listing of Items</u>

When similar items are sold, they are often placed in tables or charts for the consumer's convenience. Either scanning horizontally across a row or vertically down a column (or a combination of both) provides the opportunity for a quick comparison. Basic math plays a part in the decision making, but consumers should also consider warranties, product reputations, and hidden costs, such as tax or shipping.

For example, consider menus. Meals are individually labeled or multiple items are grouped under one heading, such as appetizers or main dishes. Substitutions may or may not have an added cost. Drinks might be ordered separately or included with the meal. Some restaurants offer free refills while others charge for each glass. If in doubt, ask your server. Regardless of the order, sales tax or a tip is seldom included. If gratuity is included, it's usually due to the size of your party and is noted on the menu. A 15-20 percent tip is customary in the United States.

For movie listings, however, prices may fluctuate based on age (teenager versus senior citizen) and time (early-bird showing versus evening). Movie listings are typically oriented vertically, either on a marquis, a display, or an easel. The current movies are usually listed with each of their show times.

Here's an example of information you could get from a menu:

since 2001

THE TOWER
MENU

Side Dishes

French Fries	$1.29
Grilled Vegetables	$1.49
Veggies Potato	$1.29
Frilled Flat Mushrooms	$2.29
Rustic Bread and Butter	$1.00
Side Combo	$2.49

(garlic and herb breaded mushrooms battered onion rings and cheesy garlic bread)

Burgers & SANDWICHES

Toast Sandwich With Smoked Salmon	$3.75
(lolo rossa, smoked salmon, horseradish, toast)	
Sandwich With Ham and Cheese	$3.35
(sexsame roll, butter, cheese, ham, salad, tomatoes, cucumber)	
Ham Sandwich	$3.35
(bavarian roll, butter, cheese, smoked ham, salad, tomatoes, cucumber)	
Sandwich Pepperoni	$3.95
(integral roll, ham, sour cream, rocked salad, cucumber)	
Mozzarella Sandwich	$3.35
(Byzantine roll, pesto sauce, mozzarella cheese, tomatoes, salad)	
Cheeseburger	$4.35
Double Cheeseburger	$6.95
Hamburger	$4.95

All of our Burgers include Pickles, Tomato Sauce and your choice of Lettuce, Tomato and Grilled Onions

BUFFET Lunch $10.95 Dinner $15.95

MAIN MEAL

Meat Mix	$9.95
(chicken fillet 60g, chicken drum stick 100g, minced meat 60g, sausage 60g, french fries, garnish)	
Homemade Sausage	$8.25
(sausage 240g, french fries, garnish)	
Grilled Chicken Fillet	$7.49
(chicken fillet 180g, french fries, garnish)	
Chicken Skewers in Bacon	$7.95
(chicken fillet 180g, 60g bacon, french fries, garnish)	
Chicken Skewers in Yoghurt Marinade	$7.25
(chicken fillet 180g, french fries, garnish)	
Baked Chicken	$7.45
(chicken fillet 180g, cheese, garnish, neutral cream, chicken fillet)	
Marinated Chicken Wings	$7.45
(chicken wings 280g, french fries, garnish)	
Chicken Drumstick	$10.00
(chicken drum stick 240g, french fries, garnish)	
Marinated Pork Neck	$8.35
(pork neck 180g, french fries, garnish)	
Chicken Fillet With Spinach and Mozzarella	$8.75
(chicken fillet 240g, french fries, garnish, mozzarella, spinach)	
Chicken Fillet With Vegetable Salad	$7.95
(chicken fillet 180g, combination of salad and mixed vegetables)	
Three Types of Meat Skewers	$9.35
(pork neck 60g, chicken fillet 60g, minced meat 60g, somun, salad mix)	
T-bone Steak	$9.95
Children's Menu	$5.35
(minced meat 100g, french fries)	

• Any additional items requested on the side will be charged at its side order price.
• Any substitution may increase the price

SALADS

Caesar Salad	$5.95
(grilled chicken, iceberg salad, crispy bacon, Caesar dressing, croutons) Add chicken breast, salmon fillet or prawns for only $1.99	
Tuna Salad	$5.95
(tuna, mix salad, corn, paprika, tomatoes, vinaigret dressing)	
Mozzarella With Prosciutto	$5.25
(prosciutto, mozzarella, paprika, tomatoes, mix salad, honey dressing)	
Choices From Salad Bar	$2.95
tomatoes, cucumber, green salad mix, sweet corn, cabage, carrot, beans, olives, two types of dressing)	

DESSERTS

Lemon ice box pie	$2.50
Boston cream pie	$2.50
Cheesecake	$2.95
Coconut cake	$2.95
Chocolate ice cream cake	$2.95

BEVERAGES and COFFEE

FREE Refill on Coffee, Iced Tea, Soft Drinks and Hot Tea

Soft Drinks	$1.49
Ice Tea	$1.49
Orange Juice	$1.49
Lemonade	$1.49
Hot Tea	$1.35
Classic Coffee	$1.35
Cappuccino	$1.50
Decaf	$1.50

Notice the various text features that make it easy to read:

- a *title* at the top to let you know what the document is for
- *headings* such as "Main Meal" and "Desserts" to help you quickly find the section you need
- different *colors*, in this case different shades of grey, to help the reader differentiate between sections
- clear, consistent *layout* with menu items on the left and prices on the right

Integration of Knowledge and Ideas

Identifying Primary Sources in Various Media

Primary sources are best defined as records or items that serve as evidence of periods of history. To be considered primary, the source documents or objects must have been created during the time period in which they reference. Examples include diaries, newspaper articles, speeches, government documents, photographs, and historical artifacts. In today's digital age, primary sources, which were once in print, often are embedded in secondary sources. Secondary sources, such as websites, history books, databases, or reviews, contain analysis or commentary on primary sources. Secondary sources borrow information from primary sources through the process of quoting, summarizing, or paraphrasing.

Today's students often complete research online through electronic sources. Electronic sources offer advantages over print, and can be accessed on virtually any computer, where libraries or other research centers are limited to fixed locations and specific catalogs. Electronic sources also are efficient and yield massive amounts of data in seconds. The user can tailor a search based on key words, publication years, and article length. Lastly, many databases provide the user with instant citations, saving the user the trouble of manually assembling sources.

Though electronic sources yield powerful results, researchers must use caution. While there are many reputable and reliable sources on the internet, just as many are unreliable or biased sources. It's up to the researcher to examine and verify the reliability of sources. *Wikipedia*, for example, may or may not be accurate, depending on the contributor. Many databases, such as *EBSCO* or *SIRS*, offer peer reviewed articles, meaning the publications have been reviewed for the quality of their content.

Using Evidence from Text to Make Predictions and Inferences, and Draw Conclusions about a Piece of Writing

Predictions
Some texts use suspense and foreshadowing to captivate readers. For example, an intriguing aspect of murder mysteries is that the reader is never sure of the culprit until the author reveals the individual's identity. Authors often build suspense and add depth and meaning to a work by leaving clues to provide hints or predict future events in the story; this is called foreshadowing. While some instances of foreshadowing are subtle, others are quite obvious.

Inferences
Another way to read actively is to identify examples of inference within text. Making an inference requires the reader to read between the lines and look for what is *implied* rather than what is directly stated. That is, using information that is known from the text, the reader is able to make a logical assumption about information that is *not* directly stated but is probably true.

Authors employ literary devices such as tone, characterization, and theme to engage the audience by showing details of the story instead of merely telling them. For example, if an author said *Bob is selfish*, there's little left to infer. If the author said, *Bob cheated on his test, ignored his mom's calls, and parked illegally*, the reader can infer Bob is selfish. Authors also make implications through character dialogue, thoughts, effects on others, actions, and looks. Like in life, readers must assemble all the clues to form a complete picture.

Read the following passage:

> "Hey, do you wanna meet my new puppy?" Jonathan asked.
>
> "Oh, I'm sorry but please don't—" Jacinta began to protest, but before she could finish, Jonathan had already opened the passenger side door of his car and a perfect white ball of fur came bouncing towards Jacinta.
>
> "Isn't he the cutest?" beamed Jonathan.
>
> "Yes—achoo!—he's pretty—aaaachooo!!—adora—aaa—aaaachoo!" Jacinta managed to say in between sneezes. "But if you don't mind, I—I—achoo!—need to go inside."

Which of the following can be inferred from Jacinta's reaction to the puppy?
   a. she hates animals
   b. she is allergic to dogs
   c. she prefers cats to dogs
   d. she is angry at Jonathan

An inference requires the reader to consider the information presented and then form their own idea about what is probably true. Based on the details in the passage, what is the best answer to the question? Important details to pay attention to include the tone of Jacinta's dialogue, which is overall polite and apologetic, as well as her reaction itself, which is a long string of sneezes. Answer choices (a) and (d) both express strong emotions ("hates" and "angry") that are not evident in Jacinta's speech or actions. Answer choice (c) mentions cats, but there is nothing in the passage to indicate Jacinta's feelings about cats. Answer choice (b), "she is allergic to dogs," is the most logical choice—based on the fact that she began sneezing as soon as a fluffy dog approached her, it makes sense to guess that Jacinta might be allergic to dogs. So even though Jacinta never directly states, "Sorry, I'm allergic to dogs!" using the clues in the passage, it is still reasonable to guess that this is true.

Making inferences is crucial for readers of literature, because literary texts often avoid presenting complete and direct information to readers about characters' thoughts or feelings, or they present this information in an unclear way, leaving it up to the reader to interpret clues given in the text. In order to make inferences while reading, readers should ask themselves:

- What details are being presented in the text?
- Is there any important information that seems to be missing?
- Based on the information that the author *does* include, what else is probably true?
- Is this inference reasonable based on what is already known?

Conclusions

Active readers should also draw conclusions. When doing so, the reader should ask the following questions: What is this piece about? What does the author believe? Does this piece have merit? Do I believe the author? Would this piece support my argument? The reader should first determine the author's intent. Identify the author's viewpoint and connect relevant evidence to support it. Readers may then move to the most important step: deciding whether to agree and determining whether they are correct. Always read cautiously and critically. Interact with text, and record reactions in the margins. These active reading skills help determine not only what the author thinks, but what the you as the reader thinks.

Comparing and Contrasting Themes from Print and Other Sources

Identifying Theme or Central Message

The *theme* is the central message of a fictional work, whether that work is structured as prose, drama, or poetry. It is the heart of what an author is trying to say to readers through the writing, and theme is largely conveyed through literary elements and techniques.

In literature, a theme can be often be determined by considering the over-arching narrative conflict with the work. Though there are several types of conflicts and several potential themes within them, the following are the most common:

- Individual against the self—relevant to themes of self-awareness, internal struggles, pride, coming of age, facing reality, fate, free will, vanity, loss of innocence, loneliness, isolation, fulfillment, failure, and disillusionment

- Individual against nature— relevant to themes of knowledge vs. ignorance, nature as beauty, quest for discovery, self-preservation, chaos and order, circle of life, death, and destruction of beauty

- Individual against society— relevant to themes of power, beauty, good, evil, war, class struggle, totalitarianism, role of men/women, wealth, corruption, change vs. tradition, capitalism, destruction, heroism, injustice, and racism

- Individual against another individual— relevant to themes of hope, loss of love or hope, sacrifice, power, revenge, betrayal, and honor

For example, in Hawthorne's *The Scarlet Letter*, one possible narrative conflict could be the individual against the self, with a relevant theme of internal struggles. This theme is alluded to through characterization—Dimmesdale's moral struggle with his love for Hester and Hester's internal struggles with the truth and her daughter, Pearl. It's also alluded to through plot—Dimmesdale's suicide and Hester helping the very townspeople who initially condemned her.

Sometimes, a text can convey a *message* or *universal lesson*—a truth or insight that the reader infers from the text, based on analysis of the literary and/or poetic elements. This message is often presented as a statement. For example, a potential message in Shakespeare's *Hamlet* could be "Revenge is what ultimately drives the human soul." This message can be immediately determined through plot and characterization in numerous ways, but it can also be determined through the setting of Norway, which is bordering on war.

How Authors Develop Theme

Authors employ a variety of techniques to present a theme. They may compare or contrast characters, events, places, ideas, or historical or invented settings to speak thematically. They may use analogies, metaphors, similes, allusions, or other literary devices to convey the theme. An author's use of diction, syntax, and tone can also help convey the theme. Authors will often develop themes through the development of characters, use of the setting, repetition of ideas, use of symbols, and through contrasting value systems. Authors of both fiction and nonfiction genres will use a variety of these techniques to develop one or more themes.

Regardless of the literary genre, there are commonalities in how authors, playwrights, and poets develop themes or central ideas.

Authors often do research, the results of which contributes to theme. In prose fiction and drama, this research may include real historical information about the setting the author has chosen or include elements that make fictional characters, settings, and plots seem realistic to the reader. In nonfiction, research is critical since the information contained within this literature must be accurate and, moreover, accurately represented.

In fiction, authors present a narrative conflict that will contribute to the overall theme. In fiction, this conflict may involve the storyline itself and some trouble within characters that needs resolution. In nonfiction, this conflict may be an explanation or commentary on factual people and events.

Authors will sometimes use character motivation to convey theme, such as in the example from *Hamlet* regarding revenge. In fiction, the characters an author creates will think, speak, and act in ways that effectively convey the theme to readers. In nonfiction, the characters are factual, as in a biography, but authors pay particular attention to presenting those motivations to make them clear to readers.

Authors also use literary devices as a means of conveying theme. For example, the use of moon symbolism in Shelley's *Frankenstein* is significant as its phases can be compared to the phases that the Creature undergoes as he struggles with his identity.

The selected point of view can also contribute to a work's theme. The use of first person point of view in a fiction or non-fiction work engages the reader's response differently than third person point of view. The central idea or theme from a first person narrative may differ from a third-person limited text.

In literary nonfiction, authors usually identify the purpose of their writing, which differs from fiction, where the general purpose is to entertain. The purpose of nonfiction is usually to inform, persuade, or entertain the audience. The stated purpose of a non-fiction text will drive how the central message or theme, if applicable, is presented.

Authors identify an audience for their writing, which is critical in shaping the theme of the work. For example, the audience for J.K. Rowling's *Harry Potter* series would be different than the audience for a biography of George Washington. The audience an author chooses to address is closely tied to the purpose of the work. The choice of an audience also drives the choice of language and level of diction an author uses. Ultimately, the intended audience determines the level to which that subject matter is presented and the complexity of the theme.

Cultural Influence on Themes

Regardless of culture, place, or time, certain themes are universal to the human condition. Because all humans experience certain feelings and engage in similar experiences—birth, death, marriage, friendship, finding meaning, etc.—certain themes span cultures. However, different cultures have different norms and general beliefs concerning these themes. For example, the theme of maturing and crossing from childhood to adulthood is a global theme; however, the literature from one culture might imply that this happens in someone's twenties, while another culture's literature might imply that it happens in the early teenage years.

It's important for the reader to be aware of these differences. Readers must avoid being *ethnocentric*, which means believing the aspects of one's own culture to be superior to that of other cultures.

Evaluating an Argument and its Specific Claims

It's important to evaluate the author's supporting details to be sure that the details are credible, provide evidence of the author's point, and directly support the main idea. Though shocking statistics grab readers' attention, their use could be ineffective information in the piece. Details like this are crucial to understanding the passage and evaluating how well the author presents their argument and evidence.

Readers draw **conclusions** about what an author has presented. This helps them better understand what the writer has intended to communicate and whether they agree with what the author has offered (or not). There are a few ways to determine a logical conclusion, but careful reading is the most important. It's helpful to read a passage a few times, noting details that seem important to the piece. Sometimes, readers arrive at a conclusion that is different than what the writer intended or come up with more than one conclusion.

Evidence

It is important to distinguish between **fact and opinion** when reading a piece of writing. When an author presents **facts**, such as statistics or data, readers should be able to check those facts and make sure they are accurate. When authors use **opinion**, they are sharing their own thoughts and feelings about a subject.

Textual evidence within the details helps readers draw a conclusion about a passage. **Textual evidence** refers to information—facts and examples that support the main point. Textual evidence will likely come from outside sources and can be in the form of quoted or paraphrased material. In order to draw a conclusion from evidence, it's important to examine the credibility and validity of that evidence as well as how (and if) it relates to the main idea.

Credibility

Critical readers examine the facts used to support an author's argument. They check the facts against other sources to be sure those facts are correct. They also check the validity of the sources used to be sure those sources are credible, academic, and/or peer- reviewed. Consider that when an author uses another person's opinion to support their argument, even if it is an expert's opinion, it is still only an opinion and should not be taken as fact. A strong argument uses valid, measurable facts to support ideas. Even then, the reader may disagree with the argument as it may be rooted in their personal beliefs.

An authoritative argument may use the facts to sway the reader. In the example of global warming, many experts differ in their opinions of what alternative fuels can be used to aid in offsetting it. Because of this, a writer may choose to only use the information and expert opinion that supports their viewpoint.

Appeal to Emotion

An author's argument might also appeal to readers' emotions, perhaps by including personal stories and *anecdotes* (a short narrative of a specific event).

The next example presents an appeal to emotion. By sharing the personal anecdote of one student and speaking about emotional topics like family relationships, the author invokes the reader's empathy in asking them to reconsider the school rule.

Our school should abolish its current ban on cell phone use on campus. If they aren't able to use their phones during the school day, many students feel isolated from their loved ones. For example, last semester, one student's grandmother had a heart attack in the morning. However, because he couldn't use his cell phone, the student didn't know about his grandmother's accident until the end of the day—when she had already passed away and it was too late to say goodbye. By preventing students from contacting their friends and family, our school is placing undue stress and anxiety on students.

Counter-Arguments

If an author presents a differing opinion or a *counter-argument* in order to refute it, the reader should consider how and why this information is being presented. It is meant to strengthen the original argument and shouldn't be confused with the author's intended conclusion, but it should also be considered in the reader's final evaluation. On the contrary, sometimes authors will concede to an opposing argument by recognizing the validity the other side has to offer. A concession will allow readers to see both sides of the argument in an unbiased light, thereby increasing the credibility of the author.

Authors can also reflect **bias** if they ignore an opposing viewpoint or present their side in an unbalanced way. A strong argument considers the opposition and finds a way to refute it. Critical readers should look for an unfair or one-sided presentation of the argument and be skeptical, as a bias may be present. Even if this bias is unintentional, if it exists in the writing, the reader should be wary of the validity of the argument.

Evaluating and Integrating Data from Multiple Source in Various Formats, Including Media

Finding Relevant Information

With a wealth of information at your fingertips in this digital age, it's important to know not only the type of information you're looking for, but also in what medium you're most likely to find it. Information needs to be specific and reliable. For example, if you're repairing a car, an encyclopedia would be mostly useless. While an encyclopedia might include information about cars, an owner's manual will contain the specific information needed for repairs. Information must also be reliable or credible so that it can be trusted. A well-known newspaper may have reliable information, but a peer-reviewed journal article will have likely gone through a more rigorous check for validity. Determining bias can be helpful in determining credibility. If the information source (person, organization, or company) has something to gain from the reader forming a certain view on a topic, it's likely the information is skewed. For example, if you are trying to find the unemployment rate, the Bureau of Labor Statistics is a more credible source than a politician's speech.

Evaluating the Credibility of a Print or Digital Source

There are several additional criteria that need to be examined before using a source for a research topic.

The following questions will help determine whether a source is credible:

- Author
- Who is he or she?
- Does he or she have the appropriate credentials—e.g., M.D, PhD?
- Is this person authorized to write on the matter through his/her job or personal experiences?
- Is he or she affiliated with any known credible individuals or organizations?
- Has he or she written anything else?
- Publisher
- Who published/produced the work? Is it a well-known journal, like National Geographic, or a tabloid, like The National Enquirer?
- Is the publisher from a scholarly, commercial, or government association?
- Do they publish works related to specific fields?
- Have they published other works?
- If a digital source, what kind of website hosts the text? Does it end in .edu, .org, or .com?
- Bias
- Is the writing objective? Does it contain any loaded or emotional language?
- Does the publisher/producer have a known bias, such as Fox News or CNN?
- Does the work include diverse opinions or perspectives?
- Does the author have any known bias—e.g., Michael Moore, Bill O'Reilly, or the Pope? Is he or she affiliated with any organizations or individuals that may have a known bias—e.g., Citizens United or the National Rifle Association?
- Does the magazine, book, journal, or website contain any advertising?

- References
- Are there any references?
- Are the references credible? Do they follow the same criteria as stated above?
- Are the references from a related field?
- Accuracy/reliability
- Has the article, book, or digital source been peer reviewed?
- Are all of the conclusions, supporting details, or ideas backed with published evidence?
- If a digital source, is it free of grammatical errors, poor spelling, and improper English?
- Do other published individuals have similar findings?
- Coverage
- Are the topic and related material both successfully addressed?
- Does the work add new information or theories to those of their sources?
- Is the target audience appropriate for the intended purpose?

Integrate Data

It's important to find multiple relevant and credible sources for data. Rather than just reading one article from a credible newspaper regarding a current event, read several articles from different newspapers. Journalists will differ in how they report a story and in which details they choose to include.

The same principle holds true for scientific or academic research. Multiple sources help give one a more thorough and balanced perspective. Be sure to find data from multiple *types* of sources as well. For instance, if you were to research the results of U.S. presidential elections it would be helpful to combine books with graphs and articles to get a comprehensive understanding.

Always consider the data from one source or type of source in light of data from our sources. A chart may convince you to think one way until you read a book that goes more into depth about the factors affecting the data.

Practice Questions

1. Xavier propagated his belief that dragons were real to his friends gathered around the campfire.
 Which of the following words could most logically replace the underlined word without altering the intent of the sentence?
    a. Shouted
    b. Expressed
    c. Persuaded
    d. Whispered

2. Which of the following statements least supports the argument that the American economy is healthy?
    a. The United States' Gross Domestic Product (GDP), which is the measure of all the goods and services produced in a country, increased by two percent last year.
    b. Unemployment is the lowest it's been in over a decade due to a spike in job creation.
    c. Average household income just hit a historical high point for the twentieth consecutive quarter.
    d. Last year, the output of the United States' manufacturing sector decreased despite repeated massive investments by both the private and public sectors.

The next three questions are based on the following table. The Dewey Decimal System is a library classification system.

The Dewey Decimal Classes
000 Computer science, information, and general works
100 Philosophy and psychology
200 Religion
300 Social sciences
400 Languages
500 Science and mathematics
600 Technical and applied science
700 Arts and recreation
800 Literature
900 History, geography, and biography

3. Teddy has been assigned to write a history paper about the United States during the Cold War. His teacher advised him to read some of the works of Noam Chomsky, an American linguist, philosopher, social scientist, cognitive scientist, historian, social critic, and political activist. Teddy was not sure where to begin, so he consulted the Dewey Decimal classes. While not all inclusive, what choice of three classes would likely be the most useful?
    a. 100, 300, 700
    b. 100, 300, 800
    c. 100, 400, 900
    d. 200, 300, 900

4. While researching Chomsky's many theories and arguments, Teddy became interested in post-World War II anarchism, a social science theory asserting the political philosophy that rejects a compulsory government. He wants to find the most appropriate works related to the subject. Which section of the library is the most likely to contain the relevant books?
   a. 000
   b. 200
   c. 300
   d. 900

5. Also during his research, Teddy discovered information about Chomsky's Jewish heritage, and he wants to research traditional Judaism as practiced in the early twentieth century. Which section of the library would most likely contain the most relevant information?
   a. 100
   b. 200
   c. 300
   d. 900

6. Which of the following statements best describes Samuel's sample size?
   a. The sample is biased because he has firsthand experience and personal knowledge of its participants.
   b. The sample contains too few members to make meaningful claims applicable to a large group.
   c. The sample contains too many members to understand the context and specifics of any given student's situation.
   d. The sample is unbiased and appropriately sized to draw conclusions on the role of parental supervision in education.

The next question is based on the following passage.

Annabelle Rice started having trouble sleeping. Her biological clock was suddenly amiss and she began to lead a nocturnal schedule. She thought her insomnia was due to spending nights writing a horror story, but then she realized that even the idea of going outside into the bright world scared her to bits. She concluded she was now suffering from heliophobia.

7. Which of the following most accurately describes the meaning of the underlined word in the sentence above?
   a. Fear of dreams
   b. Fear of sunlight
   c. Fear of strangers
   d. Anxiety spectrum disorder

The next question is based on the following directions.

Follow these instructions in chronological order to transform the word into something new.
   1. Start with the word LOATHING.
   2. Eliminate the first and last letter in the starting word.
   3. Eliminate all the vowels, except I, from the word.
   4. Eliminate the letter H from the word.

8. What new word has been spelled?
   a. TON
   b. THIN
   c. TIN
   d. TAN

9. Which of these descriptions gives the most detailed and objective support for the claim that drinking and driving is unsafe?
   a. A dramatized television commercial reenacting a fatal drinking and driving accident, including heart-wrenching testimonials from loved ones
   b. The Department of Transportation's press release noting the additional drinking and driving special patrol units that will be on the road during the holiday season
   c. Congressional written testimony on the number of drinking and driving incidents across the country and their relationship to underage drinking statistics, according to experts
   d. A highway bulletin warning drivers of penalties associated with drinking and driving

The next question is based on the following passage.

A famous children's author recently published a historical fiction novel under a pseudonym; however, it did not sell as many copies as her children's books. In her earlier years, she had majored in history and earned a graduate degree in Antebellum American History, which is the time frame of her new novel. Critics praised this newest work far more than the children's series that made her famous. In fact, her new novel was nominated for the prestigious Albert J. Beveridge Award, but still isn't selling like her children's books, which fly off the shelves because of her name alone.

10. Which one of the following statements might be accurately inferred based on the above passage?
   a. The famous children's author produced an inferior book under her pseudonym.
   b. The famous children's author is the foremost expert on Antebellum America.
   c. The famous children's author did not receive the bump in publicity for her historical novel that it would have received if it were written under her given name.
   d. People generally prefer to read children's series than historical fiction.

The next four questions are based on the following passage.

Smoking is Terrible
Smoking tobacco products is terribly destructive. A single cigarette contains over 4,000 chemicals, including 43 known carcinogens and 400 deadly toxins. Some of the most dangerous ingredients include tar, carbon monoxide, formaldehyde, ammonia, arsenic, and DDT. Smoking can cause numerous types of cancer including throat, mouth, nasal cavity, esophagus, stomach, pancreas, kidney, bladder, and cervical.

Cigarettes contain a drug called nicotine, one of the most addictive substances known to man. Addiction is defined as a compulsion to seek the substance despite negative consequences. According to the National Institute of Drug Abuse, nearly 35 million smokers expressed a desire to quit smoking in 2015; however, more than 85 percent of those addicts will not achieve their goal. Almost all smokers regret picking up that first cigarette. You would be wise to learn from their mistake if you have not yet started smoking.

According to the U.S. Department of Health and Human Services, 16 million people in the United States presently suffer from a smoking-related condition and nearly nine million suffer from a serious smoking-related illness. According to the Centers for Disease Control and Prevention (CDC), tobacco products cause nearly six million deaths per year. This number is projected to rise to over eight million deaths by 2030. Smokers, on average, die ten years earlier than their nonsmoking peers.

In the United States, local, state, and federal governments typically tax tobacco products, which leads to high prices. Nicotine addicts sometimes pay more for a pack of cigarettes than for a few gallons of gas. Additionally, smokers tend to stink. The smell of smoke is all-consuming and creates a pervasive nastiness. Smokers also risk staining their teeth and fingers with yellow residue from the tar.

Smoking is deadly, expensive, and socially unappealing. Clearly, smoking is not worth the risks.

11. Which of the following best describes the passage?
    a. Narrative
    b. Persuasive
    c. Expository
    d. Technical

12. Which of the following statements most accurately summarizes the passage?
    a. Tobacco is less healthy than many alternatives.
    b. Tobacco is deadly, expensive, and socially unappealing, and smokers would be much better off kicking the addiction.
    c. In the United States, local, state, and federal governments typically tax tobacco products, which leads to high prices.
    d. Tobacco products shorten smokers' lives by ten years and kill more than six million people per year.

13. The author would be most likely to agree with which of the following statements?
    a. Smokers should only quit cold turkey and avoid all nicotine cessation devices.
    b. Other substances are more addictive than tobacco.
    c. Smokers should quit for whatever reason that gets them to stop smoking.
    d. People who want to continue smoking should advocate for a reduction in tobacco product taxes.

14. Which of the following represents an opinion statement on the part of the author?
    a. According to the Centers for Disease Control and Prevention (CDC), tobacco products cause nearly six million deaths per year.
    b. Nicotine addicts sometimes pay more for a pack of cigarettes than a few gallons of gas.
    c. They also risk staining their teeth and fingers with yellow residue from the tar.
    d. Additionally, smokers tend to stink. The smell of smoke is all-consuming and creates a pervasive nastiness.

The next question is based on the following passage.

In 2015, 28 countries, including Estonia, Portugal, Slovenia, and Latvia, scored significantly higher than the United States on standardized high school math tests. In the 1960s, the United States consistently ranked first in the world. Today, the United States spends more than $800 billion dollars on education, which exceeds the next highest country by more than $600 billion dollars. The United States also leads the world in spending per school-aged child by an enormous margin.

15. If these statements above are factual, which of the following statements must be correct?
    a. Outspending other countries on education has benefits beyond standardized math tests.
    b. The United States' education system is corrupt and broken.
    c. The standardized math tests are not representative of American academic prowess.
    d. Spending more money does not guarantee success on standardized math tests.

16. At the top of an encyclopedia's page are the following two guide terms: kingcraft and klieg light. Which one of the following words will be found on this page?
    a. Kleptomania
    b. Knead
    c. Kinesthesia
    d. Kickback

17. Which of the following is a primary source?
    a. A critic's summary and review of a new book on the life of Abraham Lincoln
    b. A peer-reviewed scientific journal's table of contents
    c. A report containing the data, summary, and conclusions of a recent gene splicing study
    d. A news article quoting recent groundbreaking research into curing cancer

The next question is based on the following passage.

Cynthia keeps to a strict vegetarian diet, which is part of her religion. She absolutely cannot have any meat or fish dishes. This is more than a preference; her body has never developed the enzymes to process meat or fish, so she becomes violently ill if she accidentally eats any of the offending foods.

Cynthia is attending a full day event at her college next week. When at an event that serves meals, she always likes to bring a platter of vegetarian food for herself and to share with other attendees who have similar dietary restrictions. She requested a menu in advance to determine when her platter might be most useful to vegetarians. Here is the menu:

Breakfast: Hazelnut coffee or English breakfast tea, French toast, eggs, and bacon strips
Lunch: Assorted sandwiches (vegetarian options available), French fries, and baked beans
Cocktail hour: Alcoholic beverages, fruit, and cheese
Dinner: Roasted pork loin, seared trout, and bacon-bit topped macaroni and cheese

18. If Cynthia wants to pick the meal where there would be the least options for her and fellow vegetarians, during what meal should she bring the platter?
    a. Breakfast
    b. Lunch
    c. Cocktail hour
    d. Dinner

The next three questions are based on the following passage.

George Washington emerged out of the American Revolution as an unlikely champion of liberty. On June 14, 1775, the Second Continental Congress created the Continental Army, and John Adams, serving in the Congress, nominated Washington to be its first commander. Washington fought under the British during the French and Indian War, and his experience and prestige proved instrumental to the American war effort. Washington provided invaluable leadership, training, and strategy during the Revolutionary War. He emerged from the war as the embodiment of liberty and freedom from tyranny.

After vanquishing the heavily favored British forces, Washington could have pronounced himself as the autocratic leader of the former colonies without any opposition, but he famously refused and returned to his Mount Vernon plantation. His restraint proved his commitment to the fledgling state's republicanism. Washington was later unanimously elected as the first American president. But it is Washington's farewell address that cemented his legacy as a visionary worthy of study.

In 1796, President Washington issued his farewell address by public letter. Washington enlisted his good friend, Alexander Hamilton, in drafting his most famous address. The letter expressed Washington's faith in the Constitution and rule of law. He encouraged his fellow Americans to put aside partisan differences and establish a national union. Washington warned Americans against meddling in foreign affairs and entering military alliances. Additionally, he stated his opposition to national political parties, which he considered partisan and counterproductive.

Americans would be wise to remember Washington's farewell, especially during presidential elections when politics hits a fever pitch. They might want to question the political institutions that were not planned by the Founding Fathers, such as the nomination process and political parties themselves.

19. Which of the following statements is logically based on the information contained in the passage above?
    a. George Washington's background as a wealthy landholder directly led to his faith in equality, liberty, and democracy.
    b. George Washington would have opposed America's involvement in the Second World War.
    c. George Washington would not have been able to write as great a farewell address without the assistance of Alexander Hamilton.
    d. George Washington would probably not approve of modern political parties.

20. Which of the following statements is the best description of the author's purpose in writing this passage about George Washington?
    a. To inform American voters about a Founding Father's sage advice on a contemporary issue and explain its applicability to modern times
    b. To introduce George Washington to readers as a historical figure worthy of study
    c. To note that George Washington was more than a famous military hero
    d. To convince readers that George Washington is a hero of republicanism and liberty

21. In which of the following materials would the author be the most likely to include this passage?
    a. A history textbook
    b. An obituary
    c. A fictional story
    d. A newspaper editorial

The next question is based on the following conversation between a scientist and a politician.

Scientist: Last year was the warmest ever recorded in the last 134 years. During that time period, the ten warmest years have all occurred since 2000. This correlates directly with the recent increases in carbon dioxide as large countries like China, India, and Brazil continue developing and industrializing. No longer do just a handful of countries burn massive amounts of carbon-based fossil fuels; it is quickly becoming the case throughout the whole world as technology and industry spread.

Politician: Yes, but there is no causal link between increases in carbon emissions and increasing temperatures. The link is tenuous and nothing close to certain. We need to wait for all of the data before drawing hasty conclusions. For all we know, the temperature increase could be entirely natural. I believe the temperatures also rose dramatically during the dinosaurs' time, and I do not think they were burning any fossil fuels back then.

22. What is one point on which the scientist and politician agree?
    a. Burning fossil fuels causes global temperatures to rise.
    b. Global temperatures are increasing.
    c. Countries must revisit their energy policies before it's too late.
    d. Earth's climate naturally goes through warming and cooling periods.

23. Raul is going to Egypt next month. He has been looking forward to this vacation all year. Since childhood, Raul has been fascinated with pyramids, especially the Great Pyramid of Giza, which is the oldest of the Seven Wonders of the Ancient World. According to religious custom, Egyptian royalty is buried in the tombs located within the pyramid's great labyrinths. Since it has been many years since Raul read about the pyramid's history, he wants to read a book describing how and why the Egyptians built the Great Pyramid thousands of years ago. Which of the following guides would be the best for Raul?
    a. A Beginner's Guide to Giza, a short book describing the city's best historical sites, published by the Egyptian Tourism Bureau (2015)
    b. The Life of Zahi Hawass, the autobiography of one of Egypt's most famous archaeologists who was one of the first explorers at Giza (2014)
    c. A History of Hieroglyphics, an in-depth look at how archaeologists first broke the ancient code, published by the University of Giza's famed history department (2013)
    d. Who Built the Great Pyramids?, a short summary of the latest research and theories on the ancient Egyptians' religious beliefs and archaeological skills, written by a team of leading experts in the field (2015)

The next five questions are based on the following passage.

Christopher Columbus is often credited for discovering America. This is incorrect. First, it is impossible to "discover" something where people already live; however, Christopher Columbus did explore places in the New World that were previously untouched by Europe, so the term "explorer" would be more accurate. Another correction must be made, as well: Christopher Columbus was not the first European explorer to reach the present day Americas! Rather, it was Leif Erikson who first came to the New World and contacted the natives, nearly five hundred years before Christopher Columbus.

Leif Erikson, the son of Erik the Red (a famous Viking outlaw and explorer in his own right), was born in either 970 or 980, depending on which historian you seek. His own family, though, did not raise Leif, which was a Viking tradition. Instead, one of Erik's prisoners taught Leif reading and writing, languages, sailing, and weaponry. At age 12, Leif was considered a man and returned to his family. He killed a man during a dispute shortly after his return, and the council banished the Erikson clan to Greenland.

In 999, Leif left Greenland and traveled to Norway where he would serve as a guard to King Olaf Tryggvason. It was there that he became a convert to Christianity. Leif later tried to return home with the intention of taking supplies and spreading Christianity to Greenland, however his ship was blown off course and he arrived in a strange new land: present day Newfoundland, Canada.

When he finally returned to his adopted homeland Greenland, Leif consulted with a merchant who had also seen the shores of this previously unknown land we now know as Canada. The son of the legendary Viking explorer then gathered a crew of 35 men and set sail. Leif became the first European to touch foot in the New World as he explored present-day Baffin Island and Labrador, Canada. His crew called the land Vinland since it was plentiful with grapes.

During their time in present-day Newfoundland, Leif's expedition made contact with the natives whom they referred to as Skraelings (which translates to "wretched ones" in Norse). There are several secondhand accounts of their meetings. Some contemporaries described trade between the peoples. Other accounts describe clashes where the Skraelings defeated the Viking explorers with long spears, while still others claim the Vikings dominated the natives. Regardless of the circumstances, it seems that the Vikings made contact of some kind. This happened around 1000, nearly five hundred years before Columbus famously sailed the ocean blue.

Eventually, in 1003, Leif set sail for home and arrived at Greenland with a ship full of timber.

In 1020, seventeen years later, the legendary Viking died. Many believe that Leif Erikson should receive more credit for his contributions in exploring the New World.

24. Which of the following best describes how the author generally presents the information?
    a. Chronological order
    b. Comparison-contrast
    c. Cause-effect
    d. Conclusion-premises

25. Which of the following is an opinion, rather than historical fact, expressed by the author?
    a. Leif Erikson was definitely the son of Erik the Red; however, historians debate the year of his birth.
    b. Leif Erikson's crew called the land Vinland since it was plentiful with grapes.
    c. Leif Erikson deserves more credit for his contributions in exploring the New World.
    d. Leif Erikson explored the Americas nearly five hundred years before Christopher Columbus.

26. Which of the following most accurately describes the author's main conclusion?
    a. Leif Erikson is a legendary Viking explorer.
    b. Leif Erikson deserves more credit for exploring America hundreds of years before Columbus.
    c. Spreading Christianity motivated Leif Erikson's expeditions more than any other factor.
    d. Leif Erikson contacted the natives nearly five hundred years before Columbus.

27. Which of the following best describes the author's intent in the passage?
    a. To entertain
    b. To inform
    c. To alert
    d. To suggest

28. Which of the following can be logically inferred from the passage?
    a. The Vikings disliked exploring the New World.
    b. Leif Erikson's banishment from Iceland led to his exploration of present-day Canada.
    c. Leif Erikson never shared his stories of exploration with the King of Norway.
    d. Historians have difficulty definitively pinpointing events in the Vikings' history.
    The next five questions are based on the chart following a brief introduction to the topic.

The American Civil War was fought from 1861 to 1865. It is the only civil war in American history. While the South's secession was the initiating event of the war, the conflict grew out of several issues like slavery and differing interpretations of individual state rights. General Robert E. Lee led the Confederate Army for the South for the duration of the conflict (although other generals held command positions over individual battles, as you will see below). The North employed a variety of lead generals, but Ulysses S. Grant finished the war as the victorious general. There were more American casualties in the Civil War than any other military conflict in American history.

Civil War Casualties by Battle (approximate)					
Battle	Date	Union General	Confederate General	Union Casualties	Confederate Casualties
Gettysburg	July 1863	George Meade	Robert E. Lee	23,049	28,063
Chancellorsville	May 1863	Joseph Hooker	Robert E. Lee	17,304	13,460
Shiloh	April 1862	Ulysses S. Grant	Albert Sydney Johnston	13,047	10,669
Cold Harbor	May 1864	Ulysses S. Grant	Robert E. Lee	12,737	4,595
Atlanta	July 1864	William T. Sherman	John Bell Hood	3,722	5,500

29. In which of the following battles were there more Confederate casualties than Union casualties?
    a. Cold Harbor
    b. Chancellorsville
    c. Atlanta
    d. Shiloh

30. Which one of the following battles occurred first?
    a. Cold Harbor
    b. Chancellorsville
    c. Atlanta
    d. Shiloh

31. Robert E. Lee did not lead the Confederate forces in which one of the following battles?
    a. Atlanta
    b. Chancellorsville
    c. Cold Harbor
    d. Gettysburg

32. In which of the following battles did the Union casualties exceed the Confederate casualties by the greatest number?
    a. Cold Harbor
    b. Chancellorsville
    c. Atlanta
    d. Shiloh

33. The total number of American casualties suffered at the battle of Gettysburg is about double the total number of casualties suffered at which one of the following battles?
   a. Cold Harbor
   b. Chancellorsville
   c. Atlanta
   d. Shiloh
The next two questions are based on the graphic that follows a brief introduction to the topic.

The United States Constitution directs Congress to conduct a census of the population to determine the country's population and demographic information. The United States Census Bureau carries out the survey. In 1790, then Secretary of State Thomas Jefferson conducted the first census, and the most recent U.S. census was in 2010. The next U.S. census will be the first to be issued primarily through the Internet.

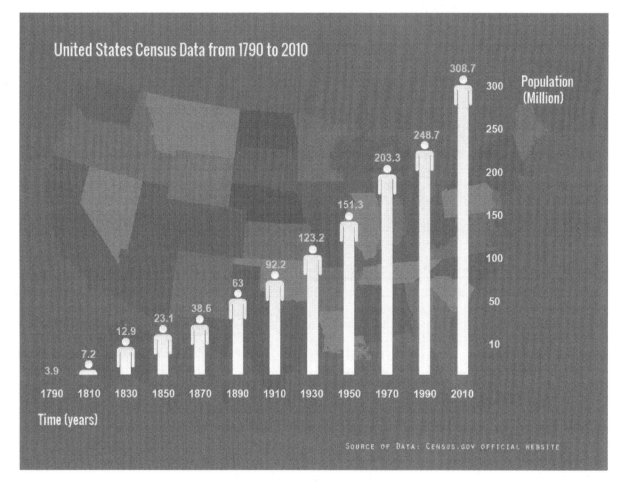

34. In which of the following years was the United States population less than it was in 1930?
   a. 1950
   b. 1970
   c. 1910
   d. 1990

35. In what year did the population increase the most during a twenty-year interval?
    a. From 1930 to 1950
    b. From 1950 to 1970
    c. From 1970 to 1990
    d. From 1990 to 2010

The next question is based on the following outline.

Chapter 5: Outdoor Activities
1. Hiking
    a. Gear
    b. First Aid
2. Camping
    a. Tents & Gear
    b. Camping Activities
3. Cycling
    a. Safety
    b. Finding Cycling Trails
4. Canoeing
    a. Equipment
    b. Tips for Maneuvering

36. What aspect of this outline is inconsistent?
    a. Hiking, which starts with an H, is included with activities that all start with C.
    b. There is no information about gear/equipment for cycling
    c. Rock climbing is not included in the outline.
    d. There is no section for hiking tips.

The next three questions are based on the graphic following a brief introduction to the topic.

A food chain is a diagram used by biologists to better understand ecosystems. It represents the interrelationships between different plants and animals. The energy is derived from the sun and converted into stored energy by plants through photosynthesis, which travels up the food chain. The energy returns to the ecosystem after the organisms die and decompose back into the Earth. This process is an endless cycle.

In food chains, living organisms are grouped into categories called primary producers and consumers, which come in multiple tiers. For example, secondary consumers feed on primary consumers, while tertiary consumers feed on secondary consumers. Apex predators are the animals at the top of the food chain. They are the highest category consumer in an ecosystem, and apex predators do not have natural predators.

37. Which of the following animals eats primary producers according to the food chain diagram?
    a. Cobra
    b. Gazelle
    c. Wild dog
    d. Aardvark

38. Which of the following animals has no natural predators according to the food chain diagram?
    a. Vulture
    b. Cobra
    c. Mongoose
    d. Aardvark

39. Which of the following is something that the mongoose would eat?
    a. Shrub
    b. Aardvark
    c. Vulture
    d. Mouse

The next four questions are based on the timeline of the life of Alexander Graham Bell.

40. Which of the following is the event that occurred fourth on the timeline?
    a. Helped found National Geographic Society
    b. Developed a metal detector
    c. Moved to Canada
    d. Started a school for the deaf

41. Of the pairings in the answer choices, which has the longest gap between the two events?
    a. Moved to Canada and Became friends with Helen Keller
    b. Became friends with Helen Keller and Died in Canada
    c. Started school for the deaf and Developed a metal detector
    d. Born in Scotland and Started school for the deaf

42. Which one of the following statements is accurate based on the timeline?
    a. Bell did nothing significant after he helped found the National Geographic Society.
    b. Bell started a school for the deaf in Canada.
    c. Bell lived in at least two countries.
    d. Developing a metal detector allowed Bell to meet Helen Keller.

43. Which one of the following events occurred most recently?
    a. Bell's invention of the telephone
    b. Bell's founding of the school.
    c. Bell's birth
    d. Bell's move to Canada

44. Which of the following statements would make the best conclusion to an essay about civil rights activist Rosa Parks?

   a. On December 1, 1955, Rosa Parks refused to give up her bus seat to a white passenger, setting in motion the Montgomery bus boycott.

   b. Rosa Parks was a hero to many, and came to symbolize the way that ordinary people could bring about real change in the Civil Rights Movement.

   c. Rosa Parks died in 2005 in Detroit, having moved from Montgomery shortly after the bus boycott.

   d. Rosa Parks' arrest was an early part of the Civil Rights Movement, and helped lead to the passage of the Civil Rights Act of 1964.

45. The following exchange occurred after the Baseball Coach's team suffered a heartbreaking loss in the final inning.

Reporter: The team clearly did not rise to the challenge. I'm sure that getting zero hits in twenty at-bats with runners in scoring position hurt the team's chances at winning the game. What are your thoughts on this devastating loss?

Baseball Coach: Hitting with runners in scoring position was not the reason we lost this game. We made numerous errors in the field, and our pitchers gave out too many free passes. Also, we did not even need a hit with runners in scoring position. Many of those at-bats could have driven in the run by simply making contact. Our team did not deserve to win the game.

Which of the following best describes the main point of dispute between the reporter and baseball coach?

   a. Whether the loss was heartbreaking.

   b. Whether getting zero hits in twenty at-bats with runners in scoring position caused the loss.

   c. Numerous errors in the field and pitchers giving too many free passes caused the loss.

   d. Whether the team deserved to win the game.

46. Read the following poem. Which option best expresses the symbolic meaning of the "road" and the overall theme?

> Two roads diverged in a yellow wood,
> And sorry I could not travel both
> And be one traveler, long I stood
> And looked down one as far as I could
> To where it bent in the undergrowth;
> Then took the other, as just as fair,
> And having perhaps the better claim,
> Because it was grassy and wanted wear;
> Though as for that the passing there
> Had worn them really about the same,
> And both that morning equally lay
> In leaves no step had trodden black.
> Oh, I kept the first for another day!
> Yet knowing how way leads on to way,
> I doubted if I should ever come back.
> I shall be telling this with a sigh
> Somewhere ages and ages hence:
> Two roads diverged in a wood, and I—
> I took the one less traveled by,
> And that has made all the difference—Robert Frost, "The Road Not Taken"

    a. A divergent spot where the traveler had to choose the correct path to his destination
    b. A choice between good and evil that the traveler needs to make
    c. The traveler's struggle between his lost love and his future prospects
    d. Life's journey and the choices with which humans are faced

47. Kimmy is a world famous actress. Millions of people downloaded her leaked movie co-starring her previous boyfriend. Kimmy earns millions through her television show and marketing appearances. There's little wonder that paparazzi track her every move.

What is the argument's primary purpose?
    a. Kimmy does not deserve her fame.
    b. Kimmy starred in an extremely popular movie.
    c. Kimmy earns millions of dollars through her television show and marketing appearances.
    d. Kimmy is a highly compensated and extremely popular television and movie actress.

48. Dwight works at a mid-sized regional tech company. He approaches all tasks with unmatched enthusiasm and leads the company in annual sales. The top salesman is always the best employee. Therefore, Dwight is the best employee.

Which of the following most accurately describes how the argument proceeds?
a. The argument proceeds by first stating a conclusion and then offering several premises to justify that conclusion.
b. The argument proceeds by stating a universal rule and then proceeds to show how this situation is the exception.
c. The argument proceeds by stating several facts that serve as the basis for the conclusion at the end of the argument.
d. The argument proceeds by stating several facts, offering a universal rule, and then drawing a conclusion by applying the facts to the rule.

Questions 49-51 are based upon the following passage:

This excerpt is adaptation from "The 'Hatchery' of the Sun-Fish"--- *Scientific American, #711*

> I have thought that an example of the intelligence (instinct?) of a class of fish which has come under my observation during my excursions into the Adirondack region of New York State might possibly be of interest to your readers, especially as I am not aware that any one except myself has noticed it, or, at least, has given it publicity.
>
> The female sun-fish (called, I believe, in England, the roach or bream) makes a "hatchery" for her eggs in this wise. Selecting a spot near the banks of the numerous lakes in which this region abounds, and where the water is about 4 inches deep, and still, she builds, with her tail and snout, a circular embankment 3 inches in height and 2 thick. The circle, which is as perfect a one as could be formed with mathematical instruments, is usually a foot and a half in diameter; and at one side of this circular wall an opening is left by the fish of just sufficient width to admit her body.
>
> The mother sun-fish, having now built or provided her "hatchery," deposits her spawn within the circular inclosure, and mounts guard at the entrance until the fry are hatched out and are sufficiently large to take charge of themselves. As the embankment, moreover, is built up to the surface of the water, no enemy can very easily obtain an entrance within the inclosure from the top; while there being only one entrance, the fish is able, with comparative ease, to keep out all intruders.
>
> I have, as I say, noticed this beautiful instinct of the sun-fish for the perpetuity of her species more particularly in the lakes of this region; but doubtless the same habit is common to these fish in other waters.

49. What is the purpose of this passage?
a. To show the effects of fish hatcheries on the Adirondack region
b. To persuade the audience to study Ichthyology (fish science)
c. To depict the sequence of mating among sun-fish
d. To enlighten the audience on the habits of sun-fish and their hatcheries

50. What does the word *wise* in this passage most closely mean?
   a. Knowledge
   b. Manner
   c. Shrewd
   d. Ignorance

51. What is the definition of the word *fry* as it appears in the following passage?
   The mother sun-fish, having now built or provided her "hatchery," deposits her spawn within the circular inclosure, and mounts guard at the entrance until the fry are hatched out and are sufficiently large to take charge of themselves.

   a. Fish at the stage of development where they are capable of feeding themselves.
   b. Fish eggs that have been fertilized.
   c. A place where larvae is kept out of danger from other predators.
   d. A dish where fish is placed in oil and fried until golden brown.

52. Read the following passage:

Write a short story with one detail in the wrong place. Maybe 5 or so sentence long.

Last week, we adopted a dog from the local animal shelter, after looking for our perfect pet for several months. We wanted a dog that was not too old, but also past the puppy stage, so that training would be less time-intensive and to give an older animal a home. Robin, as she's called, was a perfect match and we filled out our application and upon approval, were permitted to bring her home. Her physical exam and lab work all confirmed she was healthy. We went to the pet store and bought all sorts of bedding, food, toys, and treats to outfit our house as a dog-friendly and fun place. The shelter told us she liked dry food only, which is a relief because wet food is expensive and pretty off-putting. We even got fencing and installed a dog run in the backyard for Robin to roam unattended. Then we took her to the vet to make sure she was healthy. Next week, she starts the dog obedience class that we enrolled her in with a discount coupon from the shelter. It will be a good opportunity to bond with her and establish commands and dominance. When we took her to the park the afternoon after we adopted her, it was clear that she is a sociable and friendly dog, easily playing cohesively with dogs of all sizes and dispositions.

Which of the following is out of sequence in the story?
   a. Last week, we adopted a dog from the local animal shelter, after looking for our perfect pet for several months.
   b. Robin, as she's called, was a perfect match and we filled out our application and upon approval, were permitted to bring her home.
   c. Her physical exam and lab work all confirmed she was healthy.
   d. Next week, she starts the dog obedience class that we enrolled her in with a discount coupon from the shelter.

53. You are a high school math teacher and one of your students, Marcus, emailed asking to come see you after the latest exam. His email said he was disappointed and surprised with his grade and wanted to inquire about extra credit work to recoup points he lost on the exam. You decided to look over the details of his performance in your course to suss out any potential causes for his poor marks and to offer him informed tips to improve for the next exam. Thankfully, you keep detailed records to tracks each student's grades. You have four pieces of information to evaluate before he comes in to meet with you: a graph of his scores on the four exams he's taken so far, a graph of the number of absences he's had each week thus far in the course, a graph of the percentage of homework assignments he's completed each week, and an email from his basketball coach.

> From: William Cooper, Boys Varsity Basketball Coach
> To: All academic teachers
> Re: Marco
>
> Marco will be competing in the Northeast Regional Basketball tournament next week and will be absent from classes Tuesday through Friday. The student athletes will be responsible for obtaining their assignments and making arrangements to complete any missed material. If you have any questions, please don't hesitate to reach out to me. While I understand that this is not ideal so close to final exams, but this is the first time our Ravens have made it so far in the tournament and we are excited to see how well they will perform.
>
> Thanks,
> Coach William Cooper

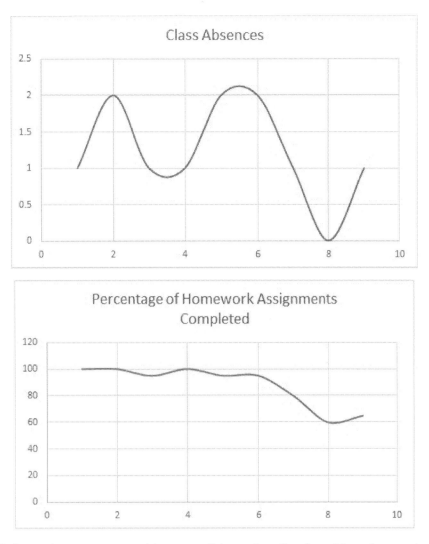

Class Absences

Percentage of Homework Assignments Completed

Which of the given information sources provides a possible explanation for a Marco's recent poor exam grade?
   a. The email from his basketball coach about the tournament
   b. The graph of his exam marks
   c. The graph of his class absences each week
   d. The graph of the percentage of homework assignments completed

Answer Explanations

1. B: To *propagate* means to spread, disseminate, promote, or otherwise make known an idea, thought, or belief. Xavier is clearly communicating his belief in dragons to his friends. Choices *A* and *D*, *whispered* and *shouted*, denote a lowered and raised decibel, respectively. Choice *C*, *persuaded*, means to cause someone to believe something in a convincing fashion. Although *persuaded* is a better answer than *whispered* or *shouted*, *expressed* is the best answer because *express* means to convey or communicate information. Choice *B* is the correct answer.

2. D: We are looking for the claim that is least supportive of the argument that the American economy is healthy. Choice *A* says that the GDP increased by 2% last year, which supports a claim of health. Choice *B* relays that unemployment is the lowest it's been in over a decade, a sign of a strong economy. Choice *C* states that average household income is at a historical high point. In contrast, the final choice draws a negative conclusion about the economy—a decrease in output even after investments—therefore, a declining manufacturing sector is least supportive that the economy is healthy. Choice *D* is the correct answer.

3. C: The question tells us that Noam Chomsky is a linguist, philosopher, social scientist, cognitive scientist, historian, social critic, and political activist. Choice *A* lists section 700, arts and recreation, which is not relevant. Choice *B* lists section 800, literature, which does not correspond to the answer. Choice *D* lists 200, religion, which is not applicable. Thus, Choice *C* is the correct answer since 100, 400, and 900 are areas of Chomsky's expertise: philosophy, languages, and history.

4. C: This question is asking you the best section to find information about anarchism. Choice *A* is not relevant. Anarchism is not a religion, so Choice *B* is not appropriate. Choice *D* would include history and perhaps provide some appropriate resources. However, anarchism is by nature and definition a social science; therefore, it best fits within the social science section. The correct section is 300, Choice *C*.

5. B: We are looking for the section where we would find books on Judaism, which is a religion. Choice *A* is about philosophy and psychology; this is not relevant, nor is Choice *C* which covers social sciences. Choice *D*, history, could be helpful, but overall, Judaism is a religion. Thus, Choice *B*, religion, is the correct answer.

6. B: Samuel wants to write an academic paper based on his 24 students. His best students come from homes where parental supervision is minimal, while the worst come from parents with extensive involvement. His conclusion is counterintuitive and probably the result of a small sample size. Choices A and D having to do with bias, is not the issue, nor is Choice C. Samuel's experience with these students is not applicable to students in general; rather, it is a tiny sample size relative to the millions of school children in the United States. The correct answer is B since the sample contains too few members to make meaningful claims applicable to a large group.

7. B: The passage indicates that Annabelle has a fear of going outside into the daylight. Thus *heliophobia* must refer to a fear of bright lights or sunlight. Choice *B* is the only answer that describes this.

8. C: After removing the first and last letter, *OATHIN* remains. Next, we eliminate all the vowels, except *I*, to get *THIN*. Finally, we remove the *H* to get *TIN*; thus, Choice *C* is the correct answer.

9. C: The answer we seek has both the most detailed and objective information. Choice *A* describing a television commercial with a dramatized reenactment is not particularly detailed. Choice *B*, a notice to the public informing them of additional drinking and driving units on patrol, is not detailed and objective information. Choice *D*, a highway bulletin, does not present the type of information required. Choice *C* is the correct answer. The number of incidents and their relationship to a possible cause are both detailed and objective information.

10. C: We are looking for an inference—a conclusion that is reached on the basis of evidence and reasoning—from the passage that will likely explain why the famous children's author did not achieve her usual success with the new genre (despite the book's acclaim). Choice A is wrong because the statement is false according to the passage. Choice B is wrong because, although the passage says the author has a graduate degree on the subject, it would be an unrealistic leap to infer that she is the foremost expert on Antebellum America. Choice D is wrong because there is nothing in the passage to lead us to infer that people generally prefer a children's series to historical fiction. In contrast, Choice C can be logically inferred since the passage speaks of the great success of the children's series and the declaration that the fame of the author's name causes the children's books to "fly off the shelves." Thus, she did not receive any bump from her name since she published the historical novel under a pseudonym, and Choice C is correct.

11. B: Narrative, Choice A, means a written account of connected events. Think of narrative writing as a story. Choice C, expository writing, generally seeks to explain or describe some phenomena, whereas Choice D, technical writing, includes directions, instructions, and/or explanations. This passage is definitely persuasive writing, which hopes to change someone's beliefs based on an appeal to reason or emotion. The author is aiming to convince the reader that smoking is terrible. They use health, price, and beauty in their argument against smoking, so Choice B, persuasive, is the correct answer.

12. B: The author is clearly opposed to tobacco. He cites disease and deaths associated with smoking. He points to the monetary expense and aesthetic costs. Choice A is wrong because alternatives to smoking are not even addressed in the passage. Choice C is wrong because it does not summarize the passage but rather is just a premise. Choice D is wrong because, while these statistics are a premise in the argument, they do not represent a summary of the piece. Choice B is the correct answer because it states the three critiques offered against tobacco and expresses the author's conclusion.

13. C: We are looking for something the author would agree with, so it will almost certainly be anti-smoking or an argument in favor of quitting smoking. Choice A is wrong because the author does not speak against means of cessation. Choice B is wrong because the author does not reference other substances, but does speak of how addictive nicotine, a drug in tobacco, is. Choice D is wrong because the author certainly would not encourage reducing taxes to encourage a reduction of smoking costs, thereby helping smokers to continue the habit. Choice C is correct because the author is definitely attempting to persuade smokers to quit smoking.

14. D: Here, we are looking for an opinion of the author's rather than a fact or statistic. Choice A is wrong because quoting statistics from the Centers of Disease Control and Prevention is stating facts, not opinions. Choice B is wrong because it expresses the fact that cigarettes sometimes cost more than a few gallons of gas. It would be an opinion if the author said that cigarettes were not affordable. Choice C is incorrect because yellow stains are a known possible adverse effect of smoking. Choice D is correct as an opinion because smell is subjective. Some people might like the smell of smoke, they might not have working olfactory senses, and/or some people might not find the smell of smoke akin to "pervasive nastiness," so this is the expression of an opinion. Thus, Choice D is the correct answer.

15. D: Outspending other countries on education could have other benefits, but there is no reference to this in the passage, so Choice A is incorrect. Choice B is incorrect because the author does not mention corruption. Choice C is incorrect because there is nothing in the passage stating that the tests are not genuinely representative. Choice D is accurate because spending more money has not brought success. The United States already spends the most money, and the country is not excelling on these tests. Choice D is the correct answer.

16. A: The guide words indicate that all of the other words on the page will be found between those words when listed alphabetically. The two guide words are *kingcraft* and *klieg light*, so the correct answer will fit between the two when ordering them alphabetically. Choice *B*, *knead*, comes after *klieg light*; Choice *C*, *kinesthesia*, and Choice *D*, *kickback*, both come before *kingcraft*. The correct answer is Choice *A*, *kleptomania*.

17. C: A primary source is an artifact, document, recording, or other source of information that is created at the time under study. Think of a primary source as the original representation of the information. In contrast, secondary sources make conclusions or draw inferences based on primary sources, as well as other secondary sources. Choice *A*, therefore, a critic's summary and review of a new book is a secondary source; additionally, the book itself may be a secondary source. Choice *B*, a table of contents, is a secondary source since it refers to other information. Choice *D*, a news article quoting research, is also a secondary source. Therefore, a report of the groundbreaking research itself, Choice *C*, is correct.

18. D: Cynthia needs to select the meal with the least vegetarian options. Although the breakfast menu, Choice *A*, includes bacon, there is also coffee, tea, French toast, and eggs available. Choice *B*, lunch, includes an option for vegetarian sandwiches along with the French fries and baked beans. The cocktail hour, Choice *C*, does not contain meat or fish. In contrast, the dinner is a vegetarian's nightmare: nothing suitable is offered. Thus, dinner, Choice *D*, is the best answer.

19. D: Although Washington is from a wealthy background, the passage does not say that his wealth led to his republican ideals, so Choice *A* is not supported. Choice *B* also does not follow from the passage. Washington's warning against meddling in foreign affairs does not mean that he would oppose wars of every kind, so Choice *B* is wrong. Choice *C* is also unjustified since the author does not indicate that Alexander Hamilton's assistance was absolutely necessary. Choice *D* is correct because the farewell address clearly opposes political parties and partisanship. The author then notes that presidential elections often hit a fever pitch of partisanship. Thus, it is follows that George Washington would not approve of modern political parties and their involvement in presidential elections.

20. A: The author finishes the passage by applying Washington's farewell address to modern politics, so the purpose probably includes this application. Choice *B* is wrong because George Washington is already a well-established historical figure; furthermore, the passage does not seek to introduce him. Choice *C* is wrong because the author is not fighting a common perception that Washington was merely a military hero. Choice *D* is wrong because the author is not convincing readers. Persuasion does not correspond to the passage. Choice *A* states the primary purpose.

21. D: Choice *A* is wrong because the last paragraph is not appropriate for a history textbook. Choice *B* is false because the piece is not a notice or announcement of Washington's death. Choice *C* is clearly false because it is not fiction, but a historical writing. Choice *D* is correct. The passage is most likely to appear in a newspaper editorial because it cites information relevant and applicable to the present day, a popular format in editorials.

22. B: The scientist and politician largely disagree, but the question asks for a point where the two are in agreement. The politician would not concur that burning fossil fuels causes global temperatures to rise; thus, Choice *A* is wrong. He would not agree with Choice *C* suggesting that countries must revisit their energy policies. By inference from the given information, the scientist would likely not concur that earth's climate naturally goes through warming and cooling cycles; so Choice *D* is incorrect. However, both the scientist and politician would agree that global temperatures are increasing. The reason for this is in dispute. The politician thinks it is part of the earth's natural cycle; the scientist thinks it is from the burning of fossil fuels. However, both acknowledge an increase, so Choice *B* is the correct answer.

23. D: Raul wants a book that describes how and why ancient Egyptians built the Great Pyramid of Giza. Choice *A* is incorrect because it focuses more generally on Giza as a whole, rather than the Great Pyramid itself. Choice *B* is close but incorrect because it is an autobiography that will largely focus on the archaeologist's life. Choice *C* is wrong because it focuses on hieroglyphics; it is not directly on point. Choice *D*, the book directly covering the building of the Great Pyramids, should be most helpful.

24. D: The passage does not proceed in chronological order since it begins by pointing out Leif Erikson's explorations in America so Choice *A* does not work. Although the author compares and contrasts Erikson with Christopher Columbus, this is not the main way the information is presented; therefore, Choice *B* does not work. Neither does Choice *C* because there is no mention of or reference to cause and effect in the passage. However, the passage does offer a conclusion (Leif Erikson deserves more credit) and premises (first European to set foot in the New World and first to contact the natives) to substantiate Erikson's historical importance. Thus, Choice *D* is correct.

25. C: Choice *A* is wrong because it describes facts: Leif Erikson was the son of Erik the Red and historians debate Leif's date of birth. These are not opinions. Choice *B* is wrong; that Erikson called the land Vinland is a verifiable fact as is Choice *D* because he did contact the natives almost 500 years before Columbus. Choice *C* is the correct answer because it is the author's opinion that Erikson deserves more credit. That, in fact, is his conclusion in the piece, but another person could argue that Columbus or another explorer deserves more credit for opening up the New World to exploration. Rather than being an incontrovertible fact, it is a subjective value claim.

26. B: Choice *A* is wrong because the author aims to go beyond describing Erikson as a mere legendary Viking. Choice *C* is wrong because the author does not focus on Erikson's motivations, let alone name the spreading of Christianity as his primary objective. Choice *D* is wrong because it is a premise that Erikson contacted the natives 500 years before Columbus, which is simply a part of supporting the author's conclusion. Choice *B* is correct because, as stated in the previous answer, it accurately identifies the author's statement that Erikson deserves more credit than he has received for being the first European to explore the New World.

27. B: Choice *A* is wrong because the author is not in any way trying to entertain the reader. Choice *D* is wrong because he goes beyond a mere suggestion; "suggest" is too vague. Although the author is certainly trying to alert the readers (make them aware) of Leif Erikson's underappreciated and unheralded accomplishments, the nature of the writing does not indicate the author would be satisfied with the reader merely knowing of Erikson's exploration (Choice *C*). Rather, the author would want the reader to be informed about it, which is more substantial (Choice *B*).

28. D: Choice *A* is wrong because the author never addresses the Vikings' state of mind or emotions. Choice *B* is wrong because the author does not elaborate on Erikson's exile and whether he would have become an explorer if not for his banishment. Choice *C* is wrong because there is not enough information to support this premise. It is unclear whether Erikson informed the King of Norway of his finding. Although it is true that the King did not send a follow-up expedition, he could have simply chosen not to expend the resources after receiving Erikson's news. It is not possible to logically infer whether Erikson told him. Choice *D* is correct because there are two examples—Leif Erikson's date of birth and what happened during the encounter with the natives—of historians having trouble pinning down important dates in Viking history.

29. C: The question asks which of the battles in the chart that are listed in this question had more Confederate casualties than Union casualties. There were more Confederate casualties than Union casualties at the Battles of Gettysburg and Atlanta. Of the two, only Atlanta is listed as an answer choice. Thus, C, Atlanta, is the correct answer.

30. D: The question is asking you to find where the dates are located in the table and to identify the earliest battle. Answer D, Shiloh, occurred in April 1862 and no other battle listed on the table happened until May 1863.

31. A: Robert E. Lee led the Confederate army in all battles listed on the table, except Shiloh and Atlanta. Shiloh is not listed in the question, therefore Atlanta, option A, is the correct answer.

32. A: This question is asking you to compare the Union and Confederate casualties and find the one listed where the Union casualties most exceeded the Confederate ones. At Cold Harbor, there were approximately 8,142 more Union casualties than Confederate. At Chancellorsville, there were approximately 3,844 more Union casualties. At Atlanta the number of Confederate casualties exceeded the Union number, so it cannot be the correct answer. At Shiloh there were approximately 2,378 more Union casualties. Thus, the number of Union casualties most greatly exceeding the Confederate number was at Cold Harbor, making *A*, Cold Harbor, the correct answer.

33. D: To calculate the total American casualties, we combine the Union and Confederate casualties since it was a civil war with Americans on both sides. There were approximately 51,112 (Union + Confederate losses) American casualties at Gettysburg; thus, the correct answer will be a battle with approximately 25,556 casualties which is half of that number. Shiloh is the closest with a total of 23,716 casualties, making D the correct answer.

34. C: The correct answer choice is C, *1910*. There are two ways to arrive at the correct answer. You could find the four answer choices on the graph, or you could have identified that the population never dips at any point. Thus, the correct answer needs to be the only answer choice that is earlier in time than the others, Choice *C*.

35. D: The population increased the most between 1990 and 2010. The question is asking you to identify the rate of change for each interval. Between 1930 and 1950, the population increased by approximately 28 million. Between 1950 and 1970, the population increased by approximately 52 million. Between 1970 and 1990, the population increased by approximately 45 million. Between 1990 and 2010, the population increased by approximately 60 million. Thus, D is the correct answer. The slope is also the steepest in this interval, which represents its higher increase.

36. B: Choice *A* is irrelevant as Chapter 5 is for outdoor activities as a whole and not only for ones that start with a particular letter. Choice *C* brings up an omission, not a potential inconsistency; furthermore, Chapter 5 does not have to include all outdoor activities. Choice *D* points out a possible inconsistency; however, it would only be an inconsistency if all the other sections contained tips. The camping section does not contain any tips. Choice *B* is the correct answer because every segment except of cycling contains a section about equipment or gear.

37. B: Primary producers make up the base of the food chain, so the correct answer will be in the level just above: a primary consumer. The cobra, wild dog, and aardvark are all secondary consumers. The gazelle is a primary consumer, so B is the correct answer.

38. A: According to the passage preceding the food chain, the apex predators do not have natural predators. So, the question is really asking which of the answer choices is an apex predator. The cobra, mongoose, and aardvark are all secondary consumers. The vulture is an apex predator; thus, a vulture has no natural predators, making A the correct answer.

39. D: A mongoose is a secondary consumer; thus, the mongoose consumes primary consumers. The shrub is a primary producer. The aardvark is a secondary consumer. The vulture is an apex predator. The mouse is a primary consumer, so Choice *D* is the correct answer.

40. D: This question is testing whether you realize how a timeline illustrates information in chronological order from left to right. "Started school for the deaf" is fourth on the timeline from the left, which means that it is the fourth event on the timeline. Thus, Choice *D* is the correct answer.

41. B: This question is asking you to determine the length of time between the pairs of events listed as answer choices. Events in timelines are arranged proportional to time. To determine the answer to this question, one must find the largest space between two events. Visually, this can be seen between the events of befriending Helen Keller and dying in Canada. Thus, choice B is the correct answer.

42. C: This question is testing whether you can discern accurate conclusions from a timeline. Although the incorrect answer choices can seem correct, they cannot be confirmed from the information presented on the timeline. Choice *A* is incorrect; while it may be reasonable to assume that the timeline documents all major life events, we do not know for certain that Bell did not engage in any notable activities after founding the National Geographic Society. Choice *B* is incorrect because the timeline does not confirm that the school was in Canada; Bell actually started it in the United States. Choice *D* is incorrect because nothing on the timeline shows causation between the two events. According to the timeline, answer choice "C" is the only verifiable statement based on the timeline. Thus, choice C is the correct answer.

43. B: The founding of the school is the event listed farthest to the right of the events in the answer choices. This means it occurred most recently. Thus, D is the correct answer.

44. B: Choice *A*, Choice *C*, and Choice *D* all relate facts but do not present the kind of general statement that would serve as an effective summary or conclusion. Choice *B* is correct.

45. B: Choice *A* uses similar language, but it is not the main point of disagreement. The reporter calls the loss devastating, and there's no reason to believe that the coach would disagree with this assessment. Eliminate this choice.

Choice *B* is strong since both passages mention the at-bats with runners in scoring position. The reporter asserts that the team lost due to the team failing to get such a hit. In contrast, the coach identifies several other reasons for the loss, including fielding and pitching errors. Additionally, the coach disagrees that the team even needed a hit in those situations.

Choice *C* is mentioned by the coach, but not by the reporter. It is unclear whether the reporter would agree with this assessment. Eliminate this choice.

Choice *D* is mentioned by the coach but not by the reporter. It is not stated whether the reporter believes that the team deserved to win. Eliminate this choice.

Therefore, Choice *B* is the correct answer.

46. D: Choice *D* correctly summarizes Frost's theme of life's journey and the choices one makes. While Choice *A* can be seen as an interpretation, it is a literal one and is incorrect. Literal is not symbolic. Choice *B* presents the idea of good and evil as a theme, and the poem does not specify this struggle for the traveler. Choice *C* is a similarly incorrect answer. Love is not the theme.

47. D: Choice *A* is irrelevant. The argument does not address whether Kimmy deserves her fame. Eliminate this choice.

Choice *B* restates a premise. Kimmy starring in an extremely popular movie is only one piece of the argument. It is not the main purpose. Eliminate this choice.

Choice *C* also restates a premise, and it is incorrect for the same reasons as Choice *B*. Eliminate this choice.

Choice *D* accurately expresses the argument's conclusion, and it best describes the argument's primary purpose. The argument concludes that Kimmy is a world famous actress. Choice *D* is the best expression of the argument's purpose.

Therefore, Choice *D* is the correct answer.

48. D: Choice *A* is clearly incorrect. The argument does not start with a conclusion. Eliminate this choice.

Choice *B* is incorrect. Although the argument states a universal rule—the top salesman is always a company's best employee—it does not argue that Dwight is the exception. Eliminate this choice.

Choice *C* is fairly strong. The argument does state several facts and offers a conclusion based on those facts. Leave this choice for now.

Choice *D* looks extremely promising. The argument first states several facts—Dwight works at a mid-sized regional tech company and leads the company in sales—then states a rule. Lastly, the argument applies the facts to the rule and concludes that Dwight is the best employee. This is a better fit than Choice *C* since it includes the rule and its application.

Therefore, Choice *D* is the correct answer.

49. D: To enlighten the audience on the habits of sun-fish and their hatcheries. Choice *A* is incorrect because although the Adirondack region is mentioned in the text, there is no cause or effect relationships between the region and fish hatcheries depicted here. Choice *B* is incorrect because the text does not have an agenda, but rather is meant to inform the audience. Finally, Choice *C* is incorrect because the text says nothing of how sun-fish mate.

50. B: The word *wise* in this passage most closely means *manner*. Choices *A* and *C* are synonyms of *wise*; however, they are not relevant in the context of the text. Choice *D*, *ignorance*, is opposite of the word *wise*, and is therefore incorrect.

51. A: Fish at the stage of development where they are capable of feeding themselves. Even if the word *fry* isn't immediately known to the reader, the context gives a hint when it says "until the fry are hatched out and are sufficiently large to take charge of themselves."

52. C: The passage is told in chronological order, detailed the steps the family took to adopt their dog. The narrator mentions that Robin's physical exam and lab work confirmed she was healthy before discussing that they brought her to the vet to evaluate her health. It is illogical that lab work would confirm good health prior to an appointment with the vet, when presumably, the lab work would be collected.

53. D: The graph displaying the percentage of weekly homework assignments Marco completed clearly shows a recent decline. It is likely that test performance may suffer without adequate practice, which is one of the primary purposes of homework assignments. Choice *A*, the email, would not necessarily substantiate a poor mark because the absences have not yet occurred and therefore, would not factor into the prior exam. Choice *B*, the graph of test scores simply demonstrates that indeed his score was lower than it had been. Choice *C* is also incorrect because his absences have no obvious trend that would lend to decreased performance. They seem to have bounced around over the duration of the course.

Mathematics

Number and Algebra

Numbers usually serve as an adjective representing a quantity of objects. They function as placeholders for a value. Numbers can be better understood by their type and related characteristics.

Definitions

A few definitions:

Whole numbers – describes a set of numbers that does not contain any fractions or decimals. The set of whole numbers includes zero.

Example: 0, 1, 2, 3, 4, 189, 293 are all whole numbers.

Integers – describes whole numbers and their negative counterparts. (Zero does not have a negative counterpart here. Instead, zero is its own negative.)

Example: -1, -2, -3, -4, -5, 0, 1, 2, 3, 4, 5 are all integers.

-1, -2, -3, -4, -5 are considered negative integers and 1, 2, 3, 4, 5 are considered positive integers.

Absolute value – describes the value of a number regardless of its sign. The symbol for absolute value is $|\,|$.

Example: The absolute value of 24 is 24 or $|24| = 24$.

The absolute value of -693 is 693 or $|-693| = 693$.

Even numbers – describes any number that can be divided evenly, meaning the answer has no decimal or remainder portion.

Example: 2, 4, 9082, -2, -16, -504 are all considered even numbers, because they can be divided by 2, without a remainder or decimal. It does not matter whether the number is positive or negative.

Odd numbers – describes any number that does not divide evenly by 2.

Example: 1, 21, 541, 3003, -9, -63, -1257 are all considered odd numbers, because they cannot be divided by 2 without a remainder or a decimal.

Prime numbers – describes a number that is only evenly divisible, resulting in no remainder or decimal, by 1 and itself.

Example: 1, 3, 9, 13, 113, -61, -11, -1 are all considered prime numbers, because they can only be evenly divided by 1 and itself.

Composite numbers – describes a positive integer that is formed by multiplying two smaller integers together. Composite numbers can be divided evenly by numbers other than 1 or itself.

Example: 24, 66, 2348, 10002 are all considered composite numbers, because they are the result of multiplying two smaller integers together. In particular, these are all divisible by 2.

Decimals - designated by a decimal point which indicates that what follows the point is a value that is less than 1 and is added to the integer number preceding the decimal point. The digit immediately following the decimal point is in the tenths place, the digit following the tenths place is in the hundredths place, and so on.

For example, the decimal number 1.735 has a value greater than 1 but less than 2. The 7 represents seven tenths of the unit 1 (0.7 or $\frac{7}{10}$); the 3 represents three hundredths of 1 (0.03 or $\frac{3}{100}$); and the 5 represents five thousandths of 1 (0.005 or $\frac{5}{1000}$).

Real numbers – describes rational numbers and irrational numbers.

Rational numbers – describes any number that can be expressed as a fraction, with a non-zero denominator. Since any integer can be written with 1 in the denominator without changing its value, all integers are considered rational numbers. Every rational number has a decimal expression that terminates or repeats. That is, any rational number either will have a countable number of nonzero digits or will end with an ellipses or a bar (3.6666... or $3.\overline{6}$) to depict repeating decimal digits. Some examples of rational numbers include 12, -3.54, $110.\overline{256}$, $\frac{-35}{10}$, and $4.\overline{7}$.

Irrational numbers – describes real numbers, which cannot be written as a finite decimal. Pi (π) is considered to be an irrational number because its decimal portion is unending or a non-repeating decimal. The most common irrational number is π, which has an endless and non-repeating decimal, but there are other well-known irrational numbers like e and $\sqrt{2}$.

Factorization

Factors are the numbers multiplied to achieve a product. Thus, every product in a multiplication equation has, at minimum, two factors. Of course, some products will have more than two factors. For the sake of most discussions, assume that factors are positive integers.

To find a number's factors, start with 1 and the number itself. Then divide the number by 2, 3, 4, and so on, seeing if any divisors can divide the number without a remainder, keeping a list of those that do. Stop upon reaching either the number itself or another factor.

Let's find the factors of 45. Start with 1 and 45. Then try to divide 45 by 2, which fails. Now divide 45 by 3. The answer is 15, so 3 and 15 are now factors. Dividing by 4 doesn't work, and dividing by 5 leaves 9. Lastly, dividing 45 by 6, 7, and 8 all don't work. The next integer to try is 9, but this is already known to be a factor, so the factorization is complete. The factors of 45 are 1, 3, 5, 9, 15 and 45.

Prime Factorization
Prime factorization involves an additional step after breaking a number down to its factors: breaking down the factors until they are all prime numbers. A prime number is any number that can be divided by 1 and itself. The prime numbers between 1 and 20 are 2, 3, 5, 7, 11, 13, 17, and 19. As a simple test, numbers that are even or end in 5 are not prime.

Let's break 129 down into its prime factors. First, the factors are 3 and 43. Both 3 and 43 are prime numbers, so we're done. But if 43 was not a prime number, then it would also need to be factorized until all of the factors are expressed as prime numbers.

Common Factor

A common factor is a factor shared by two numbers. Let's take 45 and 30 and find the common factors:

The factors of 45 are: 1, 3, 5, 9, 15, and 45.
The factors of 30 are: 1, 2, 3, 5, 6, 10, 15, and 30.
The common factors are 1, 3, 5, and 15.

Greatest Common Factor

The greatest common factor is the largest number among the shared, common factors. From the factors of 45 and 30, the common factors are 3, 5, and 15. Thus, 15 is the greatest common factor, as it's the largest number.

Least Common Multiple

The least common multiple is the smallest number that's a multiple of two numbers. Let's try to find the least common multiple of 4 and 9. The multiples of 4 are 4, 8, 12, 16, 20, 24, 28, 32, 36, and so on. For 9, the multiples are 9, 18, 27, 36, 45, 54, etc. Thus, the least common multiple of 4 and 9 is 36, the lowest number where 4 and 9 share multiples.

If two numbers share no factors besides 1 in common, then their least common multiple will be simply their product. If two numbers have common factors, then their least common multiple will be their product divided by their greatest common factor. This can be visualized by the formula $LCM = \frac{x \times y}{GCF}$, where x and y are some integers and LCM and GCF are their least common multiple and greatest common factor, respectively.

Converting Among Non-Negative Fractions, Decimals, and Percentages

Fractions

A fraction is an equation that represents a part of a whole, but can also be used to present ratios or division problems. An example of a fraction is $\frac{x}{y}$. In this example, x is called the numerator, while y is the denominator. The numerator represents the number of parts, and the denominator is the total number of parts. They are separated by a line or slash. In simple fractions, the numerator and denominator can be nearly any integer. However, the denominator of a fraction can never be zero, because dividing by zero is a function which is undefined.

Imagine that an apple pie has been baked for a holiday party, and the full pie has eight slices. After the party, there are five slices left. How could the amount of the pie that remains be expressed as a fraction? The numerator is 5 since there are 5 pieces left, and the denominator is 8 since there were eight total slices in the whole pie. Thus, expressed as a fraction, the leftover pie totals $\frac{5}{8}$ of the original amount.

Fractions come in three different varieties: proper fractions, improper fractions, and mixed numbers. Proper fractions have a numerator less than the denominator, such as $\frac{3}{8}$, but improper fractions have a numerator greater than the denominator, such as $\frac{15}{8}$. Mixed numbers combine a whole number with a proper fraction, such as $3\frac{1}{2}$. Any mixed number can be written as an improper fraction by multiplying the integer by the denominator, adding the product to the value of the numerator, and dividing the sum by the original denominator. For example:

$$3\frac{1}{2} = \frac{3 \times 2 + 1}{2} = \frac{7}{2}$$

Whole numbers can also be converted into fractions by placing the whole number as the numerator and making the denominator 1. For example, $3 = \frac{3}{1}$.

One of the most fundamental concepts of fractions is their ability to be manipulated by multiplication or division. This is possible since $\frac{n}{n} = 1$ for any non-zero integer. As a result, multiplying or dividing by $\frac{n}{n}$ will not alter the original fraction since any number multiplied or divided by 1 doesn't change the value of that number. Fractions of the same value are known as equivalent fractions. For example, $\frac{2}{4}, \frac{4}{8}, \frac{50}{100}$, and $\frac{75}{150}$ are equivalent, as they all equal $\frac{1}{2}$.

Although many equivalent fractions exist, they are easier to compare and interpret when reduced or simplified. The numerator and denominator of a simple fraction will have no factors in common other than 1. When reducing or simplifying fractions, divide the numerator and denominator by the greatest common factor. A simple strategy is to divide the numerator and denominator by low numbers, like 2, 3, or 5 until arriving at a simple fraction, but the same thing could be achieved by determining the greatest common factor for both the numerator and denominator and dividing each by it. Using the first method is preferable when both the numerator and denominator are even, end in 5, or are obviously a multiple of another number. However, if no numbers seem to work, it will be necessary to factor the numerator and denominator to find the GCF. Let's look at examples:

1) Simplify the fraction $\frac{6}{8}$:

Dividing the numerator and denominator by 2 results in $\frac{3}{4}$, which is a simple fraction.

2) Simplify the fraction $\frac{12}{36}$:

Dividing the numerator and denominator by 2 leaves $\frac{6}{18}$. This isn't a simple fraction, as both the numerator and denominator have factors in common. Diving each by 3 results in $\frac{2}{6}$, but this can be further simplified by dividing by 2 to get $\frac{1}{3}$. This is the simplest fraction, as the numerator is 1. In cases like this, multiple division operations can be avoided by determining the greatest common factor between the numerator and denominator.

3) Simplify the fraction $\frac{18}{54}$ by dividing by the greatest common factor:

First, determine the factors for the numerator and denominator. The factors of 18 are 1, 2, 3, 6, 9, and 18. The factors of 54 are 1, 2, 3, 6, 9, 18, 27, and 54. Thus, the greatest common factor is 18. Dividing $\frac{18}{54}$ by 18 leaves $\frac{1}{3}$, which is the simplest fraction. This method takes slightly more work, but it definitively arrives at the simplest fraction.

A ratio is a comparison between the relative sizes of two parts of a whole, separated by a colon. It's different from a fraction because, in a ratio, the second number represents the number of parts which aren't currently being referenced, while in a fraction, the second or bottom number represents the total number of parts in the whole. For example, if 3 pieces of an 8-piece pie were eaten, the number of uneaten parts expressed as a ratio to the number of eaten parts would be 5:3.

Equivalent ratios work just like equivalent fractions. For example, let's find two ratios equivalent to 1:3. Both 3:9 and 20:60 are equivalent ratios because both can be simplified to 1:3.

Operations with Fractions

Of the four basic operations that can be performed on fractions, the one which involves the least amount of work is multiplication. To multiply two fractions, simply multiply the numerators, multiply the denominators, and place the products as a fraction. Whole numbers and mixed numbers can also be expressed as a fraction, as described above, to multiply with a fraction. Let's work through a couple of examples.

$$1) \frac{2}{5} \times \frac{3}{4} = \frac{6}{20} = \frac{3}{10}$$

$$2) \frac{4}{9} \times \frac{7}{11} = \frac{28}{99}$$

Dividing fractions is similar to multiplication with one key difference. To divide fractions, flip the numerator and denominator of the second fraction, and then proceed as if it were a multiplication problem:

$$1) \frac{7}{8} \div \frac{4}{5} = \frac{7}{8} \times \frac{5}{4} = \frac{35}{32}$$

$$2) \frac{5}{9} \div \frac{1}{3} = \frac{5}{9} \times \frac{3}{1} = \frac{15}{9} = \frac{5}{3}$$

Addition and subtraction require more steps than multiplication and division, as these operations require the fractions to have the same denominator, also called a common denominator. It is always possible to find a common denominator by multiplying the denominators. However, when the denominators are large numbers, this method is unwieldy, especially if the answer must be provided in its simplest form. Thus, it's beneficial to find the least common denominator of the fractions—the least common denominator is incidentally also the least common multiple.

Once equivalent fractions have been found with common denominators, simply add or subtract the numerators to arrive at the answer:

$$1) \frac{1}{2} + \frac{3}{4} = \frac{2}{4} + \frac{3}{4} = \frac{5}{4}$$

$$2) \frac{3}{12} + \frac{11}{20} = \frac{15}{60} + \frac{33}{60} = \frac{48}{60} = \frac{4}{5}$$

$$3) \frac{7}{9} - \frac{4}{15} = \frac{35}{45} - \frac{12}{45} = \frac{23}{45}$$

$$4) \frac{5}{6} - \frac{7}{18} = \frac{15}{18} - \frac{7}{18} = \frac{8}{18} = \frac{4}{9}$$

Recognizing Equivalent Fractions and Mixed Numbers

The value of a fraction does not change if multiplying or dividing both the numerator and the denominator by the same number (other than 0). In other words, $\frac{x}{y} = \frac{a \times x}{a \times y} = \frac{x \div a}{y \div a}$, as long as a is not 0. This means that $\frac{2}{5} = \frac{4}{10}$, for example. If x and y are integers that have no common factors, then the fraction is said to be *simplified*. This means $\frac{2}{5}$ is simplified, but $\frac{4}{10}$ is not.

Often when working with fractions, the fractions need to be rewritten so that they all share a single denominator—this is called finding a *common denominator* for the fractions. Using two fractions, $\frac{a}{b}$ and $\frac{c}{d}$, the numerator and denominator of the left fraction can be multiplied by d, while the numerator and denominator of the right fraction can be multiplied by b. This provides the fractions $\frac{a \times d}{b \times d}$ and $\frac{c \times b}{d \times b}$ with the common denominator $b \times d$.

A fraction whose numerator is smaller than its denominator is called a *proper fraction*. A fraction whose numerator is bigger than its denominator is called an *improper fraction*. These numbers can be rewritten as a combination of integers and fractions, called a *mixed number*. For example:

$$\frac{6}{5} = \frac{5}{5} + \frac{1}{5} = 1 + \frac{1}{5}$$

It can be written as $1\frac{1}{5}$.

<u>Percentages</u>
Think of percentages as fractions with a denominator of 100. In fact, percentage means "per hundred." Problems often require converting numbers from percentages, fractions, and decimals. The following explains how to work through those conversions.

Converting Fractions to Percentages: Convert the fraction by using an equivalent fraction with a denominator of 100. For example:

$$\frac{3}{4} = \frac{3}{4} \times \frac{25}{25} = \frac{75}{100} = 75\%$$

Converting Percentages to Fractions: Percentages can be converted to fractions by turning the percentage into a fraction with a denominator of 100. Be wary of questions asking the converted fraction to be written in the simplest form. For example, $35\% = \frac{35}{100}$ which, although correctly written, has a numerator and denominator with a greatest common factor of 5 and can be simplified to $\frac{7}{20}$.

Percent Problems
The basic percent equation is the following:

$$\frac{is}{of} = \frac{\%}{100}$$

The placement of numbers in the equation depends on what the question asks.

<u>Example 1</u>
Find 40% of 80.

Basically, the problem is asking, "What is 40% of 80?" The 40% is the percent, and 80 is the number to find the percent "of." The equation is:

$$\frac{x}{80} = \frac{40}{100}$$

Solving the equation by cross-multiplication, the problem becomes 100x = 80(40). Solving for x gives the answer: x = 32.

Example 2
What percent of 100 is 20?

The 20 fills in the "is" portion, while 100 fills in the "of." The question asks for the percent, so that will be x, the unknown. The following equation is set up:

$$\frac{20}{100} = \frac{x}{100}$$

Cross-multiplying yields the equation 100x = 20(100). Solving for x gives the answer of 20%.

Example 3
30% of what number is 30?

The following equation uses the clues and numbers in the problem:

$$\frac{30}{x} = \frac{30}{100}$$

Cross-multiplying results in the equation 30(100) = 30x. Solving for x gives the answer x = 100.

Decimals
Recognition of Decimals
The *decimal system* is a way of writing out numbers that uses ten different numerals: 0, 1, 2, 3, 4, 5, 6, 7, 8, and 9. This is also called a "base ten" or "base 10" system. Other bases are also used. For example, computers work with a base of 2. This means they only use the numerals 0 and 1.

The *decimal place* denotes how far to the right of the decimal point a numeral is. The first digit to the right of the decimal point is in the *tenths* place. The next is the *hundredths*. The third is the *thousandths*.

So, 3.142 has a 1 in the tenths place, a 4 in the hundredths place, and a 2 in the thousandths place.

The *decimal point* is a period used to separate the *ones* place from the *tenths* place when writing out a number as a decimal.

A *decimal number* is a number written out with a decimal point instead of as a fraction, for example, 1.25 instead of $\frac{5}{4}$. Depending on the situation, it can sometimes be easier to work with fractions and sometimes easier to work with decimal numbers.

A decimal number is *terminating* if it stops at some point. It is called *repeating* if it never stops, but repeats a pattern over and over. It is important to note that every rational number can be written as a terminating decimal or as a repeating decimal.

Addition with Decimals
To add decimal numbers, each number in columns needs to be lined up by the decimal point. For each number being added, the zeros to the right of the last number need to be filled in so that each of the numbers has the same number of places to the right of the decimal. Then, the columns can be added together.

Here is an example of 2.45 + 1.3 + 8.891 written in column form:

$$2.450$$

$$1.300$$

$$+ 8.891$$

Zeros have been added in the columns so that each number has the same number of places to the right of the decimal.

Added together, the correct answer is 12.641:

$$2.450$$

$$1.300$$

$$+ 8.891$$

$$12.641$$

Subtraction with Decimals
Subtracting decimal numbers is the same process as adding decimals. Here is 7.89 – 4.235 written in column form:

$$7.890$$

$$- 4.235$$

$$3.655$$

A zero has been added in the column so that each number has the same number of places to the right of the decimal.

Multiplication with Decimals
Decimals can be multiplied as if there were no decimals points in the problem. For example, 0.5 x 1.25 can be rewritten and multiplied as 5 x 125, which equals 625.

The final answer will have the same number of decimal *points* as the total number of decimal *places* in the problem. The first number has one decimal place, and the second number has two decimal places. Therefore, the final answer will contain three decimal places:

$$0.5 \times 1.25 = 0.625$$

Division with Decimals
Dividing a decimal by a whole number entails using long division first by ignoring the decimal point. Then, the decimal point is moved the number of places given in the problem.

For example, 6.8 ÷ 4 can be rewritten as 68 ÷ 4, which is 17. There is one non-zero integer to the right of the decimal point, so the final solution would have one decimal place to the right of the solution. In this case, the solution is 1.7.

Dividing a decimal by another decimal requires changing the divisor to a whole number by moving its decimal point. The decimal place of the dividend should be moved by the same number of places as the divisor. Then, the problem is the same as dividing a decimal by a whole number.

For example, 5.72 ÷ 1.1 has a divisor with one decimal point in the denominator. The expression can be rewritten as 57.2 ÷ 11 by moving each number one decimal place to the right to eliminate the decimal. The long division can be completed as 572 ÷ 11 with a result of 52. Since there is one non-zero integer to the right of the decimal point in the problem, the final solution is 5.2.

In another example, 8 ÷ 0.16 has a divisor with two decimal points in the denominator. The expression can be rewritten as 800 ÷ 16 by moving each number two decimal places to the right to eliminate the decimal in the divisor. The long division can be completed with a result of 50.

Conversions

Decimals and Percentages: Since a percentage is based on "per hundred," decimals and percentages can be converted by multiplying or dividing by 100. Practically speaking, this always amounts to moving the decimal point two places to the right or left, depending on the conversion. To convert a percentage to a decimal, move the decimal point two places to the left and remove the % sign. To convert a decimal to a percentage, move the decimal point two places to the right and add a "%" sign. Here are some examples:

65% = 0.65
0.33 = 33%
0.215 = 21.5%
99.99% = 0.9999
500% = 5.00
7.55 = 755%

Fractions and Percentages: Remember that a percentage is a number per one hundred. So a percentage can be converted to a fraction by making the number in the percentage the numerator and putting 100 as the denominator:

$$43\% = \frac{43}{100}$$

$$97\% = \frac{97}{100}$$

Note that the percent symbol (%) kind of looks like a 0, a 1, and another 0. So think of a percentage like 54% as 54 over 100.

To convert a fraction to a percent, follow the same logic. If the fraction happens to have 100 in the denominator, you're in luck. Just take the numerator and add a percent symbol:

$$\frac{28}{100} = 28\%$$

Otherwise, divide the numerator by the denominator to get a decimal:

$$\frac{9}{12} = 0.75$$

Then convert the decimal to a percentage:

$$0.75 = 75\%$$

Another option is to make the denominator equal to 100. Be sure to multiply the numerator by the same number as the denominator. For example:

$$\frac{3}{20} \times \frac{5}{5} = \frac{15}{100}$$

$$\frac{15}{100} = 15\%$$

Fractions and Decimals: To convert a fraction to a decimal divide the denominator by the numerator:

$$\frac{5}{20} = 0.25$$

The other option is to multiply the numerator and denominator by whatever is needed to make the denominator equal to 100:

$$\frac{5}{20} \times \frac{5}{5} = \frac{25}{100}$$

When the denominator is equal to zero, the numerator can be directly made a decimal:

$$\frac{25}{100} = 0.25$$

To convert a fraction to a decimal follow the same logic:

$$0.65 = \frac{65}{100}$$

Then you can simplify if possible:

$$\frac{65}{100} = \frac{13}{20}$$

Performing Arithmetic Operations with Rational Numbers

Addition
Addition is the combination of two numbers so their quantities are added together cumulatively. The sign for an addition operation is the + symbol. For example, 9 + 6 = 15. The 9 and 6 combine to achieve a cumulative value, called a sum.

Addition holds the commutative property, which means that numbers in an addition equation can be switched without altering the result. The formula for the commutative property is a + b = b + a. Let's look at a few examples to see how the commutative property works:

$$7 = 3 + 4 = 4 + 3 = 7$$

$$20 = 12 + 8 = 8 + 12 = 20$$

Addition also holds the associative property, which means that the grouping of numbers don't matter in an addition problem. In other words, the presence or absence of parentheses is irrelevant. The formula for the associative property is (a + b) + c = a + (b + c). Here are some examples of the associative property at work:

$$30 = (6 + 14) + 10 = 6 + (14 + 10) = 30$$

$$35 = 8 + (2 + 25) = (8 + 2) + 25 = 35$$

There are set columns for addition: ones, tens, hundreds, thousands, ten-thousands, hundred-thousands, millions, and so on. To add how many units there are total, each column needs to be combined, starting from the right, or the ones column.

THOUSANDS	HUNDREDS	TENS	ONES

Every 10 units in the ones column equals one in the tens column, and every 10 units in the tens column equals one in the hundreds column, and so on.

Example: The number 5432 has 2 ones, 3 tens, 4 hundreds, and 5 thousands. The number 371 has 3 hundreds, 7 tens and 1 ones. To combine, or add, these two numbers, simply add up how many units of each column exist. The best way to do this is by lining up the columns:

The ones column adds 2 + 1 for a total (sum) of 3.

The tens column adds 3 + 7 for a total of 10; since 10 of that unit was collected, add 1 to the hundreds column to denote the total in the next column:

When adding the hundreds column this extra 1 needs to be combined, so it would be the sum of 4, 3, and 1.

$$4 + 3 + 1 = 8$$

The last, or thousands, column listed would be the sum of 5. Since there are no other numbers in this column, that is the final total.

The answer would look as follows:

Example
Find the sum of 9,734 and 895.

Set up the problem:

```
      9   7   3   4
+         8   9   5
_____
```

Total the columns:

```
      9   7   3   4
+         8   9   5
_____
  1   0   6   2   9
```

In this example, another column (ten-thousands) is added to the left of the thousands column, to denote a carryover of 10 units in the thousands column. The final sum is 10,629.

Subtraction

Subtraction is taking away one number from another, so their quantities are reduced. The sign designating a subtraction operation is the − symbol, and the result is called the difference. For example, 9 - 6 = 3. The number *6* detracts from the number *9* to reach the difference *3*.

Unlike addition, subtraction follows neither the commutative nor associative properties. The order and grouping in subtraction impact the result.

$$15 = 22 - 7 \neq 7 - 22 = -15$$

$$3 = (10 - 5) - 2 \neq 10 - (5 - 2) = 7$$

When working through subtraction problems involving larger numbers, it's necessary to regroup the numbers. Let's work through a practice problem using regrouping:

Here, it is clear that the ones and tens columns for 77 are greater than the ones and tens columns for 325. To subtract this number, borrow from the tens and hundreds columns. When borrowing from a column, subtracting 1 from the lender column will add 10 to the borrower column:

After ensuring that each digit in the top row is greater than the digit in the corresponding bottom row, subtraction can proceed as normal, and the answer is found to be 248.

Multiplication

Multiplication involves adding together multiple copies of a number. It is indicated by an ×symbol or a number immediately outside of a parentheses, e.g. 5(8-2). The two numbers being multiplied together are called factors, and their result is called a product. For example, $9 \times 6 = 54$. This can be shown alternatively by expansion of either the 9 or the 6:

$$9 \times 6 = 9 + 9 + 9 + 9 + 9 + 9 = 54$$

$$9 \times 6 = 6 + 6 + 6 + 6 + 6 + 6 + 6 + 6 + 6 = 54$$

Like addition, multiplication holds the commutative and associative properties:

$$115 = 23 \times 5 = 5 \times 23 = 115$$

$$84 = 3 \times (7 \times 4) = (3 \times 7) \times 4 = 84$$

Multiplication also follows the distributive property, which allows the multiplication to be distributed through parentheses. The formula for distribution is $a \times (b + c) = ab + ac$. This is clear after the examples:

$$45 = 5 \times 9 = 5(3 + 6) = (5 \times 3) + (5 \times 6) = 15 + 30 = 45$$

$$20 = 4 \times 5 = 4(10 - 5) = (4 \times 10) - (4 \times 5) = 40 - 20 = 20$$

For larger-number multiplication, how the numbers are lined up can ease the process. It is simplest to put the number with the most digits on top and the number with fewer digits on the bottom. If they have the same number of digits, select one for the top and one for the bottom. Line up the problem, and begin by multiplying the far right column on the top and the far right column on the bottom. If the answer to a column is more than 9, the one digit will be written below that column and the tens place digit will carry to the top of the next column to be added after those digits are multiplied. Write the answer below that column. Move to the next column to the left on the top, and multiply it by the same far right column on the bottom. Keep moving to the left one column at a time on the top number until the end.

Example
Multiply 37 × 8

Line up the numbers, placing the one with the most digits on top.

$$3 \quad 7$$
$$\times \qquad\qquad 8$$

Multiply the far right column on the top with the far right column on the bottom (7 x 8). Write the answer, 56, as below: The ones value, 6, gets recorded, the tens value, 5, is carried.

$$3^5 \quad 7$$
$$\times \qquad\qquad 8$$
$$6$$

Move to the next column left on the top number and multiply with the far right bottom (3 x 8). Remember to add any carry over after multiplying: 3 x 8 = 24, 24 + 5 = 29. Since there are no more digits on top, write the entire number below.

$$3^5 \quad 7$$
$$\times \qquad\qquad 8$$
$$2 \quad 9 \quad 6$$

The solution is 296

If there is more than one column to the bottom number, move to the row below the first strand of answers, mark a zero in the far right column, and then begin the multiplication process again with the far right column on top and the second column from the right on the bottom. For each digit in the bottom number, there will be a row of answers, each padded with the respective number of zeros on the right. Finally, add up all of the answer rows for one total number.

Example: Multiply 512 × 36.

Line up the numbers (the one with the most digits on top) to multiply.

Begin with the right column on top and the right column on bottom (2 × 6).

$$5 \quad 1 \quad 2$$
$$\times \quad 3 \quad 6$$

Move one column left on top and multiply by the far right column on the bottom (1 × 6). Add the carry over after multiplying: $1 \times 6 = 6, 6 + 1 = 7$.

$$5 \quad 1^1 \quad 2$$
$$\times \quad 3 \quad 6$$
$$7 \quad 2$$

Move one column left on top and multiply by the far right column on the bottom (5 × 6). Since this is the last digit on top, write the whole answer below.

```
        5   1   2
    ×           3   6
    3   0   7   2
```

Now to the second column on the bottom number. Starting on the far right column on the top, repeat this pattern for the next number left on the bottom (2 × 3). Write the answers below the first line of answers; remember to begin with a zero placeholder on the far right.

```
        5   1   2
    ×               3   6
    3   0   7   2
            6       0
```

Continue the pattern (1 × 3).

```
        5   1   2
    ×               3   6
    3   0   7   2
        3   6       0
```

Since this is the last digit on top, write the whole answer below.

```
        5   1   2
    ×               3   6
        3   0   7   2
    1   5   3   6   0
```

Now add the answer rows together. Pay attention to ensure they are aligned correctly.

```
                5   1   2
    ×                   3   6
            3   0   7   2
    +   1   5   3   6   0
        1   8   4   3   2
```

The solution is 18,432.

Multiplication becomes slightly more complicated when multiplying numbers with decimals. The easiest way to answer these problems is to ignore the decimals and multiply as if they were whole numbers. After multiplying the factors, place a decimal in the product. The placement of the decimal is determined by taking the cumulative number of decimal places in the factors.

For example:

$$
\begin{array}{r}
0.7 \\
\times\ 3 \\
\hline
2.1
\end{array}
\qquad
\begin{array}{r}
2.6 \\
\times\ 4.2 \\
\hline
10.92
\end{array}
\qquad
\begin{array}{r}
1.5 \\
\times\ 6.4 \\
\hline
9.60
\end{array}
$$

Let's tackle the first example. First, ignore the decimal and multiply the numbers as though they were whole numbers to arrive at a product: 21. Second, count the number of digits that follow a decimal (one). Finally, move the decimal place that many positions to the left, as the factors have only one decimal place. The second example works the same way, except that there are two total decimal places in the factors, so the product's decimal is moved two places over. In the third example, the decimal should be moved over two digits, but the digit zero is no longer needed, so it is erased and the final answer is 9.6.

<u>Division</u>
Division and multiplication are inverses of each other in the same way that addition and subtraction are opposites. The signs designating a division operation are the ÷ and / symbols. In division, the second number divides into the first.

The number before the division sign is called the dividend or, if expressed as a fraction, the numerator. For example, in $a \div b$, a is the dividend, while in $\frac{a}{b}$, a is the numerator.

The number after the division sign is called the divisor or, if expressed as a fraction, the denominator. For example, in $a \div b$, b is the divisor, while in $\frac{a}{b}$, b is the denominator.

Like subtraction, division doesn't follow the commutative property, as it matters which number comes before the division sign, and division doesn't follow the associative or distributive properties for the same reason. For example:

$$\frac{3}{2} = 9 \div 6 \neq 6 \div 9 = \frac{2}{3}$$

$$2 = 10 \div 5 = (30 \div 3) \div 5 \neq 30 \div (3 \div 5) = 30 \div \frac{3}{5} = 50$$

$$25 = 20 + 5 = (40 \div 2) + (40 \div 8) \neq 40 \div (2 + 8) = 40 \div 10 = 4$$

If a divisor doesn't divide into a dividend an integer number of times, whatever is left over is termed the remainder. The remainder can be further divided out into decimal form by using long division; however, this doesn't always give a quotient with a finite amount of decimal places, so the remainder can also be expressed as a fraction over the original divisor.

Example

Divide 1050/42 or 1050 ÷ 42.

Set up the problem with the denominator being divided into the numerator.

$$42\overline{)1050}$$

Check for divisibility into the first unit of the numerator, 1.

42 cannot go into 1, so add on the next unit in the denominator, 0.

42 cannot go into 10, so add on the next unit in the denominator, 5.

42 can be divided into 105, two times. Write the 2 over the 5 in 105 and multiply 42 x 2. Write the 84 under 105 for subtraction and note the remainder, 21 is less than 42.

$$
\begin{array}{r}
2 \\
42\overline{)1050} \\
-84 \\
\hline
21
\end{array}
$$

Drop the next digit in the numerator down to the remainder (making 21 into 210) to create a number 42 can divide into. 42 divides into 210 five times. Write the 5 over the 0 and multiply 42 × 5.

$$
\begin{array}{r}
25 \\
42\overline{)1050} \\
-84 \\
\hline
210
\end{array}
$$

Write the 210 under 210 for subtraction. The remainder is 0.

$$
\begin{array}{r}
25 \\
42\overline{)1050} \\
-84 \\
\hline
210 \\
-210 \\
\hline
0
\end{array}
$$

The solution is 25.

Example
Divide 375/4 or 375 ÷ 4.

Set up the problem.

$$4\overline{)375}$$

4 cannot divide into 3, so add the next unit from the numerator, 7. 4 divides into 37 nine times, so write the 9 above the 7. Multiply $4 \times 9 = 36$. Write the 36 under the 37 for subtraction. The remainder is 1 (1 is less than 4).

$$
\begin{array}{r}
9 \\
4\overline{)375} \\
-36 \\
\hline
1
\end{array}
$$

Drop the next digit in the numerator, 5, making the remainder 15. 4 divides into 15, three times, so write the 3 above the 5. Multiply 4×3. Write the 12 under the 15 for subtraction, remainder is 3 (3 is less than 4)

$$
\begin{array}{r}
93 \\
4\overline{)375} \\
-36 \\
\hline
15 \\
-12 \\
\hline
3
\end{array}
$$

The solution is 93 remainder 3 or 93 ¾ (the remainder can be written over the original denominator).

Division with decimals is similar to multiplication with decimals in that when dividing a decimal by a whole number, ignore the decimal and divide as if it were a whole number.

Upon finding the answer, or quotient, place the decimal at the decimal place equal to that in the dividend.

$$15.75 \div 3 = 5.25$$

When the divisor is a decimal number, multiply both the divisor and dividend by 10. Repeat this until the divisor is a whole number, then complete the division operation as described above.

$$17.5 \div 2.5 = 175 \div 25 = 7$$

Exponents
An exponent is an operation used as shorthand for a number multiplied or divided by itself for a defined number of times:

$$3^7 = 3 \times 3 \times 3 \times 3 \times 3 \times 3 \times 3$$

In this example, the 3 is called the base and the 7 is called the exponent. The exponent is typically expressed as a superscript number near the upper right side of the base, but can also be identified as the number following a caret symbol (^). This operation would be verbally expressed as "3 to the 7th power" or "3 raised to the power

74

of 7." Common exponents are 2 and 3. A base raised to the power of 2 is referred to as having been "squared," while a base raised to the power of 3 is referred to as having been "cubed."

Several special rules apply to exponents. First, the Zero Power Rule finds that any number raised to the zero power equals 1. For example, 100^0, 2^0, $(-3)^0$ and 0^0 all equal 1 because the bases are raised to the zero power.

Second, exponents can be negative. With negative exponents, the equation is expressed as a fraction, as in the following example:

$$3^{-7} = \frac{1}{3^7} = \frac{1}{3 \text{ x } 3 \text{ x } 3 \text{ x } 3 \text{ x } 3 \text{ x } 3 \text{ x } 3}$$

Third, the Power Rule concerns exponents being raised by another exponent. When this occurs, the exponents are multiplied by each other:

$$(x^2)^3 = x^6 = (x^3)^2$$

Fourth, when multiplying two exponents with the same base, the Product Rule requires that the base remains the same and the exponents are added. For example, a^xx $a^y = a^{x+y}$. Since addition and multiplication are commutative, the two terms being multiplied can be in any order.

$$x^3x^5 = x^{3+5} = x^8 = x^{5+3} = x^5x^3$$

Fifth, when dividing two exponents with the same base, the Quotient Rule requires that the base remains the same, but the exponents are subtracted. So, $a^x \div a^y = a^{x-y}$. Since subtraction and division are not commutative, the two terms must remain in order.

$$x^5x^{-3} = x^{5-3} = x^2 = x^5 \div x^3 = \frac{x^5}{x^3}$$

Additionally, 1 raised to any power is still equal to 1, and any number raised to the power of 1 is equal to itself. In other words, $a^1 = a$ and $14^1 = 14$.

Exponents play an important role in scientific notation to present extremely large or small numbers as follows: $a \times 10^b$. To write the number in scientific notation, the decimal is moved until there is only one digit on the left side of the decimal point, indicating that the number a has a value between 1 and 10. The number of times the decimal moves indicates the exponent to which 10 is raised, here represented by b. If the decimal moves to the left, then b is positive, but if the decimal moves to the right, then b is negative.

See the following examples:

$$3,050 = 3.05 \times 10^3$$

$$-777 = -7.77 \times 10^2$$

$$0.000123 = 1.23 \times 10^{-4}$$

$$-0.0525 = -5.25 \times 10^{-2}$$

Roots
The *square root symbol* is expressed as $\sqrt{\ }$ and is commonly known as the radical. Taking the root of a number is the inverse operation of multiplying that number by itself some amount of times. For example, squaring the

number 7 is equal to 7×7, or 49. Finding the square root is the opposite of finding an exponent, as the operation seeks a number that when multiplied by itself equals the number in the square root symbol.

For example, $\sqrt{36}$ = 6 because 6 multiplied by 6 equals 36. Note, the square root of 36 is also -6 since -6 x -6 = 36. This can be indicated using a plus/minus symbol like this: ±6. However, square roots are often just expressed as a positive number for simplicity with it being understood that the true value can be either positive or negative.

Perfect squares are numbers with whole number–square roots. The list of perfect squares begins with 0, 1, 4, 9, 16, 25, 36, 49, 64, 81, and 100.

Determining the square root of imperfect squares requires a calculator to reach an exact figure. It's possible, however, to approximate the answer by finding the two perfect squares that the number fits between. For example, the square root of 40 is between 6 and 7 since the squares of those numbers are 36 and 49, respectively.

Square roots are the most common root operation. If the radical doesn't have a number to the upper left of the symbol $\sqrt{\ }$, then it's a square root. Sometimes a radical includes a number in the upper left, like $\sqrt[3]{27}$, as in the other common root type—the cube root. Complicated roots like the cube root often require a calculator.

Parentheses
Parentheses separate different parts of an equation, and operations within them should be thought of as taking place before the outside operations take place. Practically, this means that the distinction between what is inside and outside of the parentheses decides the order of operations that the equation follows. Failing to solve operations inside the parentheses before addressing the part of the equation outside of the parentheses will lead to incorrect results.

For example, let's analyze $5 - (3 + 25)$. The addition operation within the parentheses must be solved first. So $3 + 25 = 28$, leaving $5 - (28) = -23$. If this was solve in the incorrect order of operations, the solution might be found to be $5 - 3 + 25 = 2 + 25 = 27$, which would be wrong.

Equations often feature multiple layers of parentheses. To differentiate them, square brackets [ ] and braces { } are used in addition to parentheses. The innermost parentheses must be solved before working outward to larger brackets. For example, in $\{2 \div [5 - (3 + 1)]\}$, solving the innermost parentheses $(3 + 1)$ leaves $\{2 \div [5 - (4)]\}$. $[5 - (4)]$ is now the next smallest, which leaves $\{2 \div [1]\}$ in the final step, and 2 as the answer.

Order of Operations
When solving equations with multiple operations, special rules apply. These rules are known as the Order of Operations. The order is as follows: Parentheses, Exponents, Multiplication and Division from left to right, and Addition and Subtraction from left to right. A popular pneumonic device to help remember the order is Please Excuse My Dear Aunt Sally (PEMDAS). Evaluate the following two problems to understand the Order of Operations:

1) $4 + (3 \times 2)^2 \div 4$

First, solve the operation within the parentheses: $4 + 6^2 \div 4$.
Second, solve the exponent: $4 + 36 \div 4$.
Third, solve the division operation: $4 + 9$.
Fourth, finish the operation with addition for the answer, 13.

2) $2 \times (6 + 3) \div (2 + 1)^2$

$\quad$ $2 \times 9 \div (3)^2$
$\quad$ $2 \times 9 \div 9$
$\quad$ $18 \div 9$
$\quad$ 2

Positive and Negative Numbers
Signs
Aside from 0, numbers can be either positive or negative. The sign for a positive number is the plus sign or the + symbol, while the sign for a negative number is minus sign or the − symbol. If a number has no designation, then it's assumed to be positive.

Absolute Values
Both positive and negative numbers are valued according to their distance from 0. Look at this number line for +3 and -3:

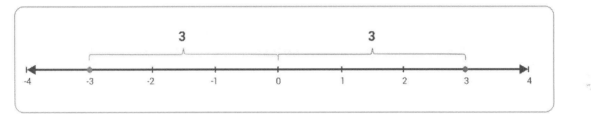

Both 3 and -3 are three spaces from 0. The distance from 0 is called its absolute value. Thus, both -3 and 3 have an absolute value of 3 since they're both three spaces away from 0.

An absolute number is written by placing | | around the number. So, $|3|$ and $|-3|$ both equal 3, as that's their common absolute value.

Implications for Addition and Subtraction
For addition, if all numbers are either positive or negative, simply add them together. For example, 4 + 4 = 8 and -4 + -4 = -8. However, things get tricky when some of the numbers are negative and some are positive.

Take 6 + (-4) as an example. First, take the absolute values of the numbers, which are 6 and 4. Second, subtract the smaller value from the larger. The equation becomes $6 - 4 = 2$. Third, place the sign of the original larger number on the sum. Here, 6 is the larger number, and it's positive, so the sum is 2.

Here's an example where the negative number has a larger absolute value: (-6) + 4. The first two steps are the same as the example above. However, on the third step, the negative sign must be placed on the sum, as the absolute value of (-6) is greater than 4. Thus, -6 + 4 = -2.

The absolute value of numbers implies that subtraction can be thought of as flip the sign of the number following the subtraction sign and simply adding the two numbers. This means that subtracting a negative number will in fact be adding the positive absolute value of the negative number. Here are some examples:

$$-6 - 4 = -6 + -4 = -10$$

$$3 - -6 = 3 + 9 = 12$$

$$-3 - 2 = -3 + -2 = -5$$

<u>Implications for Multiplication and Division</u>

For multiplication and division, if both numbers are positive, then the product or quotient is always positive. If both numbers are negative, then the product or quotient is also positive. However, if the numbers have opposite signs, the product or quotient is always negative.

Simply put, the product in multiplication and quotient in division is always positive, unless the numbers have opposing signs, in which case it's negative. Here are some examples:

$$(-6) \times (-5) = 30$$

$$(-50) \div 10 = -5$$

$$8 \times |-7| = 56$$

$$(-48) \div (-6) = 8$$

If there are more than two numbers in a multiplication problem, then whether the product is positive or negative depends on the number of negative numbers in the problem. If there is an odd number of negatives, then the product is negative. If there is an even number of negative numbers, then the result is positive.

Here are some examples:

$$(-6) \times 5 \times (-2) \times (-4) = -240$$

$$(-6) \times 5 \times 2 \times (-4) = 240$$

Comparing and Ordering Rational Numbers

A common question type asks to order rational numbers from least to greatest or greatest to least. The numbers will come in a variety of formats, including decimals, percentages, roots, fractions, and whole numbers. These questions test for knowledge of different types of numbers and the ability to determine their respective values.

Whether the question asks to order the numbers from greatest to least or least to greatest, the crux of the question is the same—convert the numbers into a common format. Generally, it's easiest to write the numbers as whole numbers and decimals so they can be placed on a number line. Follow these examples to understand this strategy.

1) Order the following rational numbers from greatest to least:

$$\sqrt{36}, 0.65, 78\%, \frac{3}{4}, 7, 90\%, \frac{5}{2}$$

Of the seven numbers, the whole number (7) and decimal (0.65) are already in an accessible form, so concentrate on the other five.

First, the square root of 36 equals 6. (If the test asks for the root of a non-perfect root, determine which two whole numbers the root lies between.) Next, convert the percentages to decimals. A percentage means "per hundred," so this conversion requires moving the decimal point two places to the left, leaving 0.78 and 0.9. Lastly, evaluate the fractions:

$$\frac{3}{4} = \frac{75}{100} = 0.75 \; ; \frac{5}{2} = 2\frac{1}{2} = 2.5$$

Now, the only step left is to list the numbers in the request order:

$$7, \sqrt{36}, \frac{5}{2}, 90\%, 78\%, \frac{3}{4}, 0.65$$

2) Order the following rational numbers from least to greatest:

$$2.5, \sqrt{9}, -10.5, 0.853, 175\%, \sqrt{4}, \frac{4}{5}$$

$$\sqrt{9} = 3$$

$$175\% = 1.75$$

$$\sqrt{4} = 2$$

$$\frac{4}{5} = 0.8$$

From least to greatest, the answer is:

$$-10.5, \frac{4}{5}, 0.853, 175\%, \sqrt{4}, 2.5, \sqrt{9}$$

Solving Equations in One Variable

Solving equations in one variable is the process of isolating a variable on one side of the equation. The letters in an equation and any numbers attached to them are the variables as they stand for unknown quantities that you are trying to solve for. X is commonly used as a variable, though any letter can be used. For example, in $3x - 7 = 20$, the variable is $3x$, and it needs to be isolated. The numbers (also called constants) are -7 and 20. That means $3x$ needs to be on one side of the equals sign (either side is fine) and all the numbers need to be on the other side of the equals sign.

To accomplish this, the equation must be manipulated by performing opposite operations of what already exists. Remember that addition and subtraction are opposites and that multiplication and division are opposites. Any action take to one side of the equation must be taken on the other side to maintain equality.

So, since the 7 is being subtracted, it can be moved to the right side of the equation by adding seven to both sides:

$$3x - 7 = 20$$

$$3x - 7 + 7 = 20 + 7$$

$$3x = 27$$

Now that the variable $3x$ is on one side and the constants (now combined into one constant) are on the other side, the 3 needs to be moved to the right side. 3 and x are being multiplied together, so 3 then needs to be divided from each side.

$$\frac{3x}{3} = \frac{27}{3}$$

$$x = 9$$

Now x has been completely isolated and thus we knows its value.

The solution is found to be $x = 9$. This solution can be checked for accuracy by plugging $x = 9$ in the original equation. After simplifying the equation, $20 = 20$ is found, which is a true statement:

$$3 \times 9 - 7 = 20$$

$$27 - 7 = 20$$

$$20 = 20$$

Equations that require solving for a variable (*algebraic equations*) come in many forms. Here are some more examples:

No number attached to the variable:

$$x + 8 = 20$$

$$x + 8 - 8 = 20 - 8$$

$$x = 12$$

Fraction in the variable:

$$\frac{1}{2}z + 24 = 36$$

$$\frac{1}{2}z + 24 - 24 = 36 - 24$$

$$\frac{1}{2}z = 12$$

Now we multiply the variable by its inverse:

$$\frac{2}{1} \times \frac{1}{2}z = 12 \times \frac{2}{1}$$

$$z = 24$$

Multiple instances of x:

$$14x + x - 4 = 3x + 2$$

All instances of x can be combined.

$$15x - 4 = 3x + 2$$

$$15x - 4 + 4 = 3x + 2 + 4$$

$$15x = 3x + 6$$

$$15x - 3x = 3x + 6 - 3x$$

$$12x = 6$$

$$\frac{12x}{12} = \frac{6}{12}$$

$$x = \frac{1}{2}$$

Solving Real Word One- or Multi-Step Problems with Rational Numbers

Word problems can appear daunting, but don't let the verbiage psyche you out. No matter the scenario or specifics, the key to answering them is to translate the words into a math problem. Always keep in mind what the question is asking and what operations could lead to that answer. The following word problems highlight the most commonly tested question types.

<u>Working with Money</u>
Walter's Coffee Shop sells a variety of drinks and breakfast treats.

Price List	
Hot Coffee	$2.00
Slow-Drip Iced Coffee	$3.00
Latte	$4.00
Muffin	$2.00
Crepe	$4.00
Egg Sandwich	$5.00

Costs	
Hot Coffee	$0.25
Slow-Drip Iced Coffee	$0.75
Latte	$1.00
Muffin	$1.00
Crepe	$2.00
Egg Sandwich	$3.00

Walter's utilities, rent, and labor costs him $500 per day. Today, Walter sold 200 hot coffees, 100 slow-drip iced coffees, 50 lattes, 75 muffins, 45 crepes, and 60 egg sandwiches. What was Walter's total profit today?

To accurately answer this type of question, determine the total cost of making his drinks and treats, then determine how much revenue he earned from selling those products. After arriving at these two totals, the profit is measured by deducted the total cost from the total revenue.

Walter's costs for today:

Item	Quantity	Cost Per Unit	Total Cost
Hot Coffee	200	$0.25	$50
Slow-Drip Iced Coffee	100	$0.75	$75
Latte	50	$1.00	$50
Muffin	75	$1.00	$75
Crepe	45	$2.00	$90
Egg Sandwich	60	$3.00	$180
Utilities, rent, and labor			$500
Total Costs			$1,020

Walter's revenue for today:

Item	Quantity	Revenue Per Unit	Total Revenue
Hot Coffee	200	$2.00	$400
Slow-Drip Iced Coffee	100	$3.00	$300
Latte	50	$4.00	$200
Muffin	75	$2.00	$150
Crepe	45	$4.00	$180
Egg Sandwich	60	$5.00	$300
Total Revenue			$1,530

Walter's Profit = *Revenue* − *Costs* = $1,530 − $1,020 = $510

This strategy is applicable to other question types. For example, calculating salary after deductions, balancing a checkbook, and calculating a dinner bill are common word problems similar to business planning. Just remember to use the correct operations. When a balance is increased, use addition. When a balance is decreased, use subtraction. Common sense and organization are your greatest assets when answering word problems.

Solving Real-World Problems Involving Percentages

Questions dealing with percentages can be difficult when they are phrased as word problems. These word problems almost always come in three varieties. The first type will ask to find what percentage of some number will equal another number. The second asks to determine what number is some percentage of another given number. The third will ask what number another number is a given percentage of.

One of the most important parts of correctly answering percentage word problems is to identify the numerator and the denominator. This fraction can then be converted into a percentage, as described above.

The following word problem shows how to make this conversion:

A department store carries several different types of footwear. The store is currently selling 8 athletic shoes, 7 dress shoes, and 5 sandals. What percentage of the store's footwear are sandals?

First, calculate what serves as the 'whole', as this will be the denominator. How many total pieces of footwear does the store sell? The store sells 20 different types (8 athletic + 7 dress + 5 sandals).

Second, what footwear type is the question specifically asking about? Sandals. Thus, 5 is the numerator.

Third, the resultant fraction must be expressed as a percentage. The first two steps indicate that $\frac{5}{20}$ of the footwear pieces are sandals. This fraction must now be converted into a percentage:

$$\frac{5}{20} \times \frac{5}{5} = \frac{25}{100} = 25\%$$

Applying Estimation Strategies and Rounding Rules to Real-World Problems

Estimation
Estimation is finding a value that is close to a solution but is not the exact answer. For example, if there are values in the thousands to be multiplied, then each value can be estimated to the nearest thousand and the calculation performed. This value provides an approximate solution that can be determined very quickly.

Rounding Numbers
It's often convenient to round a number, which means to give an approximate figure to make it easier to compare amounts or perform mental math. Round up when the digit is 5 or more. The rounded digit, and all subsequent digits, becomes 0, and the preceding digit goes up by 1. Here are some examples:

> 75 rounded to the nearest ten is 80
> 380 rounded to the nearest hundred is 400
> 22.697 rounded to the nearest hundredth is 22.70

Round down when rounding on any digit that is below 5. The rounded digit, and all subsequent digits, becomes 0, and the preceding digit goes down by 1. Here are some examples:

> 92 rounded to the nearest ten is 90
> 839 rounded to the nearest hundred is 800
> 22.643 rounded to the nearest hundredth is 22.64

Determining the Reasonableness of Results
When solving math word problems, the solution obtained should make sense within the given scenario. The step of checking the solution will reduce the possibility of a calculation error or a solution that may be *mathematically* correct but not applicable in the real world. Consider the following scenarios:

A problem states that Lisa got 24 out of 32 questions correct on a test and asks to find the percentage of correct answers. To solve the problem, a student divided 32 by 24 to get 1.33, and then multiplied by 100 to get 133 percent. By examining the solution within the context of the problem, the student should recognize that getting all 32 questions correct will produce a perfect score of 100 percent. Therefore, a score of 133 percent with 8 incorrect answers does not make sense and the calculations should be checked.

A problem states that the maximum weight on a bridge cannot exceed 22,000 pounds. The problem asks to find the maximum number of cars that can be on the bridge at one time if each car weighs 4,000 pounds. To solve this problem, a student divided 22,000 by 4,000 to get an answer of 5.5. By examining the solution within the context of the problem, the student should recognize that although the calculations are mathematically correct, the solution does not make sense. Half of a car on a bridge is not possible, so the student should determine that a maximum of 5 cars can be on the bridge at the same time.

Mental Math Estimation

Once a result is determined to be logical within the context of a given problem, the result should be evaluated by its nearness to the expected answer. This is performed by approximating given values to perform mental math. Numbers should be rounded to the nearest value possible to check the initial results.

Consider the following example: A problem states that a customer is buying a new sound system for their home. The customer purchases a stereo for $435, 2 speakers for $67 each, and the necessary cables for $12. The customer chooses an option that allows him to spread the costs over equal payments for 4 months. How much will the monthly payments be?

After making calculations for the problem, a student determines that the monthly payment will be $145.25. To check the accuracy of the results, the student rounds each cost to the nearest ten ($440 + 70 + 70 + 10$) and determines that the total is approximately $590. Dividing by 4 months gives an approximate monthly payment of $147.50. Therefore, the student can conclude that the solution of $145.25 is very close to what should be expected.

When rounding, the place-value that is used in rounding can make a difference. Suppose the student had rounded to the nearest hundred for the estimation. The result ($400 + 100 + 100 + 0 = 600;\ 600 \div 4 = 150$) will show that the answer is reasonable, but not as close to the actual value as rounding to the nearest ten.

Solving Real-World Problems Involving Proportions

Much like a scale factor can be written using an equation like $2A = B$, a *relationship* is represented by the equation $Y = kX$. X and Y are proportional because as values of X increase, the values of Y also increase. A relationship that is inversely proportional can be represented by the equation $Y = \frac{k}{x}$, where the value of Y decreases as the value of x increases and vice versa.

Proportional reasoning can be used to solve problems involving ratios, percentages, and averages. Ratios can be used in setting up proportions and solving them to find unknowns. For example, if student completes an average of 10 pages of math homework in 3 nights, how long would it take the student to complete 22 pages? Both ratios can be written as fractions. The second ratio would contain the unknown.

The following proportion represents this problem, where x is the unknown number of nights:

$$\frac{10\ pages}{3\ nights} = \frac{22\ pages}{x\ nights}$$

Solving this proportion entails cross-multiplying and results in the following equation: $10x = 22 * 3$. Simplifying and solving for x results in the exact solution: $x = 6.6\ nights$. The result would be rounded up to 7 because the homework would be actually be completed on the 7th night.

The following problem uses ratios involving percentages:

If 20% of the class is girls and 30 students are in the class, how many girls are in the class?

To set up this problem, it is helpful to use the common proportion: $\frac{\%}{100} = \frac{is}{of}$. Within the proportion, % is the percentage of girls, 100 is the total percentage of the class, *is* is the number of girls, and *of* is the total number of students in the class. Most percentage problems can be written using this language. To solve this problem, the proportion should be set up as $\frac{20}{100} = \frac{x}{30}$, and then solved for x. Cross-multiplying results in the equation $20 * 30 = 100x$, which results in the solution $x = 6$. There are 6 girls in the class.

Problems involving volume, length, and other units can also be solved using ratios. For example, a problem may ask for the volume of a cone to be found that has a radius, $r = 7m$ and a height, $h = 16m$. Referring to the formulas provided on the test, the volume of a cone is given as: $V = \pi r^2 \frac{h}{3}$, where r is the radius, and h is the height. Plugging $r = 7$ and $h = 16$ into the formula, the following is obtained: $V = \pi(7^2)\frac{16}{3}$. Therefore, volume of the cone is found to be approximately 821m³. Sometimes, answers in different units are sought. If this problem wanted the answer in liters, 821m³ would need to be converted. Using the equivalence statement 1m³ = 1000L, the following ratio would be used to solve for liters: $821m^3 * \frac{1000L}{1m^3}$. Cubic meters in the numerator and denominator cancel each other out, and the answer is converted to 821,000 liters, or $8.21 * 10^5$ L.

Other conversions can also be made between different given and final units. If the temperature in a pool is 30°C, what is the temperature of the pool in degrees Fahrenheit? To convert these units, an equation is used relating Celsius to Fahrenheit. The following equation is used: $T_{^\circ F} = 1.8T_{^\circ C} + 32$. Plugging in the given temperature and solving the equation for T yields the result: $T_{^\circ F} = 1.8(30) + 32 = 86^\circ F$. Both units in the metric system and U.S. customary system are widely used.

Here are some more examples of how to solve for proportions:

1) $\frac{75\%}{90\%} = \frac{25\%}{x}$

To solve for x, the fractions must be cross multiplied: ($75\%x = 90\% \times 25\%$). To make things easier, let's convert the percentages to decimals: ($0.9 \times 0.25 = 0.225 = 0.75x$). To get rid of x's co-efficient, each side must be divided by that same coefficient to get the answer $x = 0.3$. The question could ask for the answer as a percentage or fraction in lowest terms, which are 30% and $\frac{3}{10}$, respectively.

2) $\frac{x}{12} = \frac{30}{96}$

Cross-multiply: $96x = 30 \times 12$

Multiply: $96x = 360$

Divide: $x = 360 \div 96$

Answer: $x = 3.75$

3) $\frac{0.5}{3} = \frac{x}{6}$

Cross-multiply: $3x = 0.5 \times 6$

Multiply: $3x = 3$

Divide: $x = 3 \div 3$

Answer: $x = 1$

You may have noticed there's a faster way to arrive at the answer. If there is an obvious operation being performed on the proportion, the same operation can be used on the other side of the proportion to solve for x. For example, in the first practice problem, 75% became 25% when divided by 3, and upon doing the same to 90%, the correct answer of 30% would have been found with much less legwork. However, these questions aren't always so intuitive, so it's a good idea to work through the steps, even if the answer seems apparent from the outset.

Solving Real-World Problems Involving Ratios and Rates of Change

Ratios are used to show the relationship between two quantities. The ratio of oranges to apples in the grocery store may be 3 to 2. That means that for every 3 oranges, there are 2 apples. This comparison can be expanded to represent the actual number of oranges and apples. Another example may be the number of boys to girls in a math class. If the ration of boys to girls is given as 2 to 5, that means there are 2 boys to every 5 girls in the class. Ratios can also be compared if the units in each ratio are the same. The ratio of boys to girls in the math class can be compared to the ratio of boys to girls in a science class by stating which ratio is higher and which is lower.

Rates are used to compare two quantities with different units. *Unit rates* are the simplest form of rate. With unit rates, the denominator in the comparison of two units is one. For example, if someone can type at a rate of 1000 words in 5 minutes, then his or her unit rate for typing is $\frac{1000}{5} = 200$ words in one minute or 200 words per minute. Any rate can be converted into a unit rate by dividing to make the denominator one. 1000 words in 5 minutes has been converted into the unit rate of 200 words per minute.

Ratios and rates can be used together to convert rates into different units. For example, if someone is driving 50 kilometers per hour, that rate can be converted into miles per hour by using a ratio known as the *conversion factor*. Since the given value contains kilometers and the final answer needs to be in miles, the ratio relating miles to kilometers needs to be used. There are 0.62 miles in 1 kilometer. This, written as a ratio and in fraction form, is $\frac{0.62\ miles}{1\ km}$. To convert 50km/hour into miles per hour, the following conversion needs to be set up: $\frac{50\ km}{hour} * \frac{0.62\ miles}{1\ km} = 31\ miles\ per\ hour.$

The ratio between two similar geometric figures is called the *scale factor*. For example, a problem may depict two similar triangles, A and B. The scale factor from the smaller triangle A to the larger triangle B is given as 2 because the length of the corresponding side of the larger triangle, 16, is twice the corresponding side on the smaller triangle, 8. This scale factor can also be used to find the value of a missing side, x, in triangle A. Since the scale factor from the smaller triangle (A) to larger one (B) is 2, the larger corresponding side in triangle B (given as 25), can be divided by 2 to find the missing side in A ($x = 12.5$). The scale factor can also be represented in the equation $2A = B$ because two times the lengths of A gives the corresponding lengths of B. This is the idea behind similar triangles.

Unit Rate
Unit rate word problems will ask to calculate the rate or quantity of something in a different value. For example, a problem might say that a car drove a certain number of miles in a certain number of minutes and then ask how many miles per hour the car was traveling. These questions involve solving proportions. Consider the following examples:

86

1) Alexandra made $96 during the first 3 hours of her shift as a temporary worker at a law office. She will continue to earn money at this rate until she finishes in 5 more hours. How much does Alexandra make per hour? How much will Alexandra have made at the end of the day?

This problem can be solved in two ways. The first is to set up a proportion, as the rate of pay is constant. The second is to determine her hourly rate, multiply the 5 hours by that rate, and then add the $96.

To set up a proportion, put the money already earned over the hours already worked on one side of an equation. The other side has x over 8 hours (the total hours worked in the day). It looks like this: $\frac{96}{3} = \frac{x}{8}$. Now, cross-multiply to get $768 = 3x$. To get x, divide by 3, which leaves $x = 256$. Alternatively, as x is the numerator of one of the proportions, multiplying by its denominator will reduce the solution by one step. Thus, Alexandra will make $256 at the end of the day. To calculate her hourly rate, divide the total by 8, giving $32 per hour.

Alternatively, it is possible to figure out the hourly rate by dividing $96 by 3 hours to get $32 per hour. Now her total pay can be figured by multiplying $32 per hour by 8 hours, which comes out to $256.

2) Jonathan is reading a novel. So far, he has read 215 of the 335 total pages. It takes Jonathan 25 minutes to read 10 pages, and the rate is constant. How long does it take Jonathan to read one page? How much longer will it take him to finish the novel? Express the answer in time.

To calculate how long it takes Jonathan to read one page, divide the 25 minutes by 10 pages to determine the page per minute rate. Thus, it takes 2.5 minutes to read one page.

Jonathan must read 120 more pages to complete the novel. (This is calculated by subtracting the pages already read from the total.) Now, multiply his rate per page by the number of pages. Thus, $120 \div 2.5 = 300$. Expressed in time, 300 minutes is equal to 5 hours.

3) At a hotel, $\frac{4}{5}$ of the 120 rooms are booked for Saturday. On Sunday, $\frac{3}{4}$ of the rooms are booked. On which day are more of the rooms booked, and by how many more?

The first step is to calculate the number of rooms booked for each day. Do this by multiplying the fraction of the rooms booked by the total number of rooms.

Saturday: $\frac{4}{5} \times 120 = \frac{4}{5} \times \frac{120}{1} = \frac{480}{5} = 96$ rooms

Sunday: $\frac{3}{4} \times 120 = \frac{3}{4} \times \frac{120}{1} = \frac{360}{4} = 90$ rooms

Thus, more rooms were booked on Saturday by 6 rooms.

4) In a veterinary hospital, the veterinarian-to-pet ratio is 1:9. The ratio is always constant. If there are 45 pets in the hospital, how many veterinarians are currently in the veterinary hospital?

Set up a proportion to solve for the number of veterinarians: $\frac{1}{9} = \frac{x}{45}$

Cross-multiplying results in $9x = 45$, which works out to 5 veterinarians.

Alternatively, as there are always 9 times as many pets as veterinarians, is it possible to divide the number of pets (45) by 9. This also arrives at the correct answer of 5 veterinarians.

5) At a general practice law firm, 30% of the lawyers work solely on tort cases. If 9 lawyers work solely on tort cases, how many lawyers work at the firm?

First, solve for the total number of lawyers working at the firm, which will be represented here with x. The problem states that 9 lawyers work solely on torts cases, and they make up 30% of the total lawyers at the firm. Thus, 30% multiplied by the total, x, will equal 9. Written as equation, this is: $30\% \times x = 9$.

It's easier to deal with the equation after converting the percentage to a decimal, leaving $0.3x = 9$. Thus, $x = \frac{9}{0.3} = 30$ lawyers working at the firm.

6) Xavier was hospitalized with pneumonia. He was originally given 35mg of antibiotics. Later, after his condition continued to worsen, Xavier's dosage was increased to 60mg. What was the percent increase of the antibiotics? Round the percentage to the nearest tenth.

An increase or decrease in percentage can be calculated by dividing the difference in amounts by the original amount and multiplying by 100. Written as an equation, the formula is:

$$\frac{new\ quantity\ -\ old\ quantity}{old\ quantity} \times 100$$

Here, the question states that the dosage was increased from 35mg to 60mg, so these are plugged into the formula to find the percentage increase.

$$\frac{60\ -\ 35}{35} \times 100 = \frac{25}{35} \times 100 = .7142 \times 100 = 71.4\%$$

Rate of Change

Rate of change for any line calculates the steepness of the line over a given interval. Rate of change is also known as the slope or rise/run. The TEAS will focus on the rate of change for linear functions which are straight lines. The slope is given by the change in *y* divided by the change in *x*. So the formula looks like this:

$$slope = \frac{y_2 - y_1}{x_2 - x_1}$$

In the graph below, two points are plotted. The first has the coordinates of (0,1) and the second point is (2,3). Remember that the x coordinate is always placed first in coordinate pairs. Work from left to right when identifying coordinates. Thus the point on the left is point 1 (0,1) and the point on the right is point 2 (2,3).

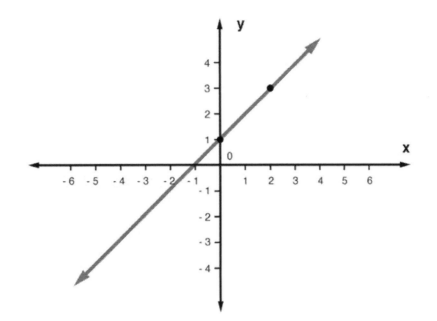

Now we need to just plug those numbers into the equation:

$$slope = \frac{3-1}{2-0}$$

$$slope = \frac{2}{2}$$

$$slope = 1$$

This means that for every increase of 1 for x, y also increased by 1. You can see this in the line. When x equalled 0, y equalled 1, and when x was increased to 1, y equalled 2.

Slope can be thought of as determining the rise over run:

$$slope = \frac{rise}{run}$$

The rise being the change vertically on the y axis and the run being the change horizontally on the x axis.

Translating Phrases and Sentences into Expressions, Equations, and Inequalities

When asked rewrite a mathematical expression as a situation or translate a word problem into an expression, look for a series of key words indicating addition, subtraction, multiplication, or division:

Addition: add, altogether, together, plus, increased by, more than, in all, sum, and total

Subtraction: minus, less than, difference, decreased by, fewer than, remain, and take away

Multiplication: *times*, *twice*, *of*, *double*, and *triple*

Division: divided by, cut up, half, quotient of, split, and shared equally

If a question asks to give words to a mathematical expression and says "equals," then an = sign must be included in the answer. Similarly, "less than or equal to" is expressed by the inequality symbol ≤, and "greater than or equal" to is expressed as ≥. Furthermore, "less than" is represented by <, and "greater than" is expressed by >.

Measurement and Data

Interpreting Relevant Information from Tables, Charts, and Graphs

Interpretation of Tables, Charts, and Graphs
Data can be represented in many ways. It is important to be able to organize the data into categories that could be represented using one of these methods. Equally important is the ability to read these types of diagrams and interpret their meaning.

Data in Tables
One of the most common ways to express data is in a table. The primary reason for plugging data into a table is to make interpretation more convenient. It's much easier to look at the table than to analyze results in a narrative paragraph. When analyzing a table, pay close attention to the title, variables, and data.

Let's analyze a theoretical antibiotic study. The study has 6 groups, named A through F, and each group receives a different dose of medicine. The results of the study are listed in the table below.

Results of Antibiotic Studies		
Group	**Dosage of Antibiotics in milligrams (mg)**	**Efficacy (% of participants cured)**
A	0 mg	20%
B	20 mg	40%
C	40 mg	75%
D	60 mg	95%
E	80 mg	100%
F	100 mg	100%

Tables generally list the title immediately above the data. The title should succinctly explain what is listed below. Here, "Results of Antibiotic Studies" informs the audience that the data pertains to the results of scientific study on antibiotics.

Identifying the variables at play is one of the most important parts of interpreting data. Remember, the independent variable is intentionally altered, and its change is independent of the other variables. Here, the dosage of antibiotics administered to the different groups is the independent variable. The study is intentionally manipulating the strength of the medicine to study the related results. Efficacy is the dependent variable since its results *depend* on a different variable, the dose of antibiotics. Generally, the independent variable will be listed before the dependent variable in tables.

Also play close attention to the variables' labels. Here, the dose is expressed in milligrams (mg) and efficacy in percentages (%). Keep an eye out for questions referencing data in a different unit measurement, as discussed in the next topic, or questions asking for a raw number when only the percentage is listed.

Now that the nature of the study and variables at play have been identified, the data itself needs be interpreted. Group A did not receive any of the medicine. As discussed earlier, Group A is the control, as it reflects the amount of people cured in the same timeframe without medicine. It's important to see that efficacy positively correlates with the dosage of medicine. A question using this study might ask for the lowest dose of antibiotics to achieve 100% efficacy. Although Group E and Group F both achieve 100% efficacy, it's important to note that Group E reaches 100% with a lower dose.

Data in Graphs

Graphs provide a visual representation of data. The variables are placed on the two axes. The bottom of the graph is referred to as the horizontal axis or X-axis. The left-hand side of the graph is known as the vertical axis or Y-axis. Typically, the independent variable is placed on the X-axis, and the dependent variable is located on the Y-axis. Sometimes the X-axis is a timeline, and the dependent variables for different trials or groups have been measured throughout points in time; time is still an independent variable, but is not always immediately thought of as the independent variable being studied.

The most common types of graphs are the bar graph and the line graph.

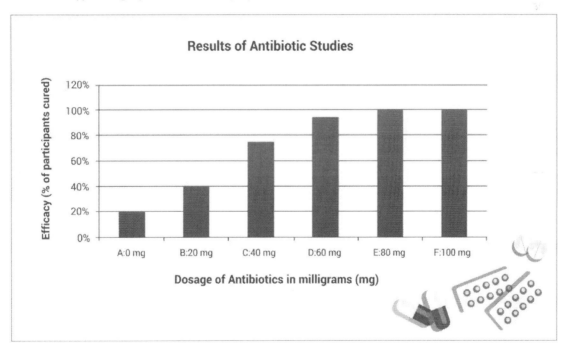

91

The *bar graph* above expresses the data from the table entitled "Results of Antibiotic Studies." To interpret the data for each group in the study, look at the top of their bars and read the corresponding efficacy on the Y-axis.

Here, the same data is expressed on a *line graph*. The points on the line correspond with each data entry. Reading the data on the line graph works like the bar graph. The data trend is be measured by the slope of the line.

Data in Other Charts

Chart is a broad term that refers to a variety of ways to represent data.

To graph relations, the *Cartesian plane* is used. This means to think of the plane as being given a grid of squares, with one direction being the *x*-axis and the other direction the *y*-axis. Generally, the independent variable is placed along the horizontal axis, and the dependent variable is placed along the vertical axis. Any point on the plane can be specified by saying how far to go along the *x*-axis and how far along the *y*-axis with a pair of numbers (x, y). Specific values for these pairs can be given names such as $C = (-1, 3)$. Negative values mean to move left or down; positive values mean to move right or up. The point where the axes cross one another is called the *origin*. The origin has coordinates $(0, 0)$ and is usually called O when given a specific label. An illustration of the Cartesian plane, along with graphs of $(2, 1)$ and $(-1, -1)$, are below.

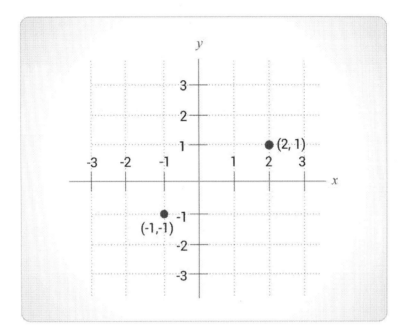

A *line plot* is a diagram that shows quantity of data along a number line. It is a quick way to record data in a structure similar to a bar graph without needing to do the required shading of a bar graph. Here is an example of a line plot:

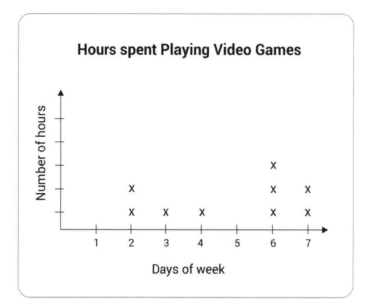

A *tally chart* is a diagram in which tally marks are utilized to represent data. Tally marks are a means of showing a quantity of objects within a specific classification. Here is an example of a tally chart:

Number of days with rain	Number of weeks
0	II
1	HHT
2	HHT
3	HHT
4	HHT HHT HHT IIII
5	HHT I
6	HHT I
7	IIII

Data is often recorded using fractions, such as half a mile, and understanding fractions is critical because of their popular use in real-world applications. Also, it is extremely important to label values with their units when using data. For example, regarding length, the number 2 is meaningless unless it is attached to a unit. Writing 2 cm shows that the number refers to the length of an object.

A *picture graph* is a diagram that shows pictorial representation of data being discussed. The symbols used can represent a certain number of objects. Notice how each fruit symbol in the following graph represents a count of two fruits. One drawback of picture graphs is that they can be less accurate if each symbol represents a large number. For example, if each banana symbol represented ten bananas, and students consumed 22 bananas, it may be challenging to draw and interpret two and one-fifth bananas as a frequency count of 22.

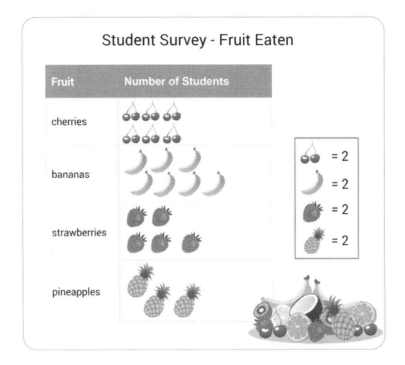

A circle graph, also called a pie chart, shows categorical data with each category representing a percentage of the whole data set. To make a circle graph, the percent of the data set for each category must be determined. To do so, the frequency of the category is divided by the total number of data points and converted to a percent. For example, if 80 people were asked what their favorite sport is and 20 responded basketball, basketball makes up 25% of the data ($\frac{20}{80}$ =.25=25%). Each category in a data set is represented by a *slice* of the circle proportionate to its percentage of the whole.

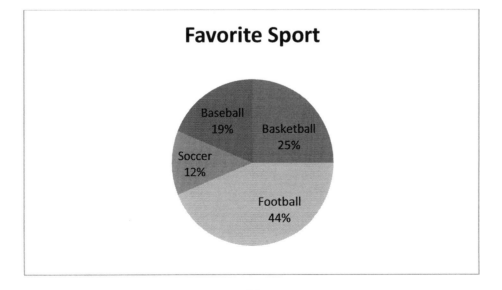

A scatter plot displays the relationship between two variables. Values for the independent variable, typically denoted by *x*, are paired with values for the dependent variable, typically denoted by *y*. Each set of corresponding values are written as an ordered pair (*x*, *y*). To construct the graph, a coordinate grid is labeled with the *x*-axis representing the independent variable and the *y*-axis representing the dependent variable. Each ordered pair is graphed.

Like a scatter plot, a line graph compares two variables that change continuously, typically over time. Paired data values (ordered pair) are plotted on a coordinate grid with the *x*- and *y*-axis representing the two variables. A line is drawn from each point to the next, going from left to right. A double line graph simply displays two sets of data that contain values for the same two variables. The double line graph below displays the profit for given years (two variables) for Company A and Company B (two data sets).

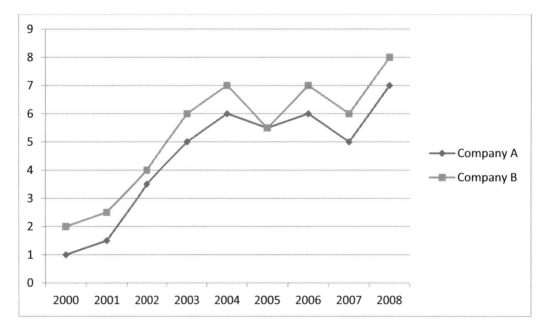

Choosing the appropriate graph to display a data set depends on what type of data is included in the set and what information must be shown.

Scatter plots and line graphs can be used to display data consisting of two variables. Examples include height and weight, or distance and time. A correlation between the variables is determined by examining the points on the graph. Line graphs are used if each value for one variable pairs with a distinct value for the other variable. Line graphs show relationships between variables.

Interpreting Competing Data

Be careful of questions with competing studies. These questions will ask to interpret which of two studies shows the greater amount or the higher rate of change between two results.

Here's an example. A research facility runs studies on two different antibiotics: Drug A and Drug B. The Drug A study includes 1,000 participants and cures 600 people. The Drug B study includes 200 participants and cures 150 people. Which drug is more successful?

The first step is to determine the percentage of each drug's rate of success. Drug A was successful in curing 60% of participants, while Drug B achieved a 75% success rate. Thus, Drug B is more successful based on these studies, even though it cured fewer people.

Sample size and experiment consistency should also be considered when answering questions based on competing studies. Is one study significantly larger than the other? In the antibiotics example, the Drug A study is five times larger than Drug B. Thus, Drug B's higher efficacy (desired result) could be a result of the smaller sample size, rather than the quality of drug.

Consistency between studies is directly related to sample size. Let's say the research facility elects to conduct more studies on Drug B. In the next study, there are 400 participants, and 200 are cured. The success rate of the second study is 50%. The results are clearly inconsistent with the first study, which means more testing is needed to determine the drug's efficacy. A hallmark of mathematical or scientific research is repeatability. Studies should be consistent and repeatable, with an appropriately large sample size, before drawing extensive conclusions.

Evaluating the Information in Tables, Charts, and Graphs Using Statistics

Mean, Median, and Mode

The center of a set of data (statistical values) can be represented by its mean, median, or mode. These are sometimes referred to as measures of central tendency.

Mean

The first property that can be defined for this set of data is the *mean*. This is the same as average. To find the mean, add up all the data points, then divide by the total number of data points. For example, suppose that in a class of 10 students, the scores on a test were 50, 60, 65, 65, 75, 80, 85, 85, 90, 100. Therefore, the average test score will be:

$$\frac{50 + 60 + 65 + 65 + 75 + 80 + 85 + 85 + 90 + 100}{10} = 75.5$$

The mean is a useful number if the distribution of data is normal (more on this later), which roughly means that the frequency of different outcomes has a single peak and is roughly equally distributed on both sides of that peak. However, it is less useful in some cases where the data might be split or where there are some *outliers*. Outliers are data points that are far from the rest of the data. For example, suppose there are 11 executives and 90 employees at a company. The executives make $1000 per hour, and the employees make $10 per hour.

Therefore, the average pay rate will be:

$$\frac{\$1000 \cdot 11 + \$10 \cdot 90}{100} = \$119 \; per \; hour$$

In this case, this average is not very descriptive since it's not close to the actual pay of the executives *or* the employees.

Median

Another useful measurement is the *median*. In a data set, the median is the point in the middle. The middle refers to the point where half the data comes before it and half comes after, when the data is recorded in numerical order. For instance, these are the speeds of the fastball of a pitcher during the last inning that he pitched (in order from least to greatest):

90, 92, 93, 93, 95, 96, 97, 97, 97

There are nine total numbers, so the middle or *median* number in the 5th one, which is 95.

In cases where the number of data points is an even number than the average of the two middle points it taken. In the previous example of test scores, the two middle points are 75 and 80. Since there is no single point, the average of these two scores needs to be found. The average is:

$$\frac{75 + 80}{2} = 77.5$$

The median is generally a good value to use if there are a few outliers in the data. It prevents those outliers from affecting the "middle" value as much as when using the mean.

Since an outlier is a data point that is far from most of the other data points in a data set, this means an outlier also is any point that is far from the median of the data set. The outliers can have a substantial effect on the mean of a data set, but usually do not change the median or mode, or do not change them by a large quantity. For example, consider the data set (3, 5, 6, 6, 6, 8). This has a median of 6 and a mode of 6, with a mean of $\frac{34}{6} \approx 5.67$. Now, suppose a new data point of 1000 is added so that the data set is now (3, 5, 6, 6, 6, 8, 1000). This does not change the median or mode, which are both still 6. However, the average is now $\frac{1034}{7}$, which is approximately 147.7. In this case, the median and mode will be better descriptions for most of the data points.

The reason for outliers in a given data set is a complicated problem. It is sometimes the result of an error by the experimenter, but often they are perfectly valid data points that must be taken into consideration.

Mode

One additional measure to define for *X* is the *mode*. This is the data point that appears most frequently. If two or more data points all tie for the most frequent appearance, then each of them is considered a mode. In the case of the test scores, where the numbers were 50, 60, 65, 65, 75, 80, 85, 85, 90, 100, there are two modes: 65 and 85.

Describing a Set of Data

A set of data can be described in terms of its center, spread, shape and any unusual features. The center of a data set can be measured by its mean, median, or mode. The spread of a data set refers to how far the data points are from the center (mean or median). A data set with data points clustered around the center will have a small spread. A data set covering a wide range will have a large spread.

When a data set is displayed as a graph like the one below, the shape indicates if a sample is normally distributed, symmetrical, or has measures of skewness. When graphed, a data set with a normal distribution will resemble a bell curve.

If the data set is symmetrical, each half of the graph when divided at the center is a mirror image of the other. If the graph has fewer data points to the right, the data is skewed right. If it has fewer data points to the left, the data is skewed left.

A description of a data set should include any unusual features such as gaps or outliers. A gap is a span within the range of the data set containing no data points. An outlier is a data point with a value either extremely large or extremely small when compared to the other values in the set.

The graphs above can be referred to as *unimodal* since they all have a single peak. This is contrast to *bimodal* graph that have multiple peaks.

<u>Correlation</u>

An *X-Y diagram*, also known as a scatter diagram, visually displays the relationship between two variables. The independent variable is placed on the *x-axis*, or horizontal axis, and the dependent variable is placed on the *y-axis*, or vertical axis.

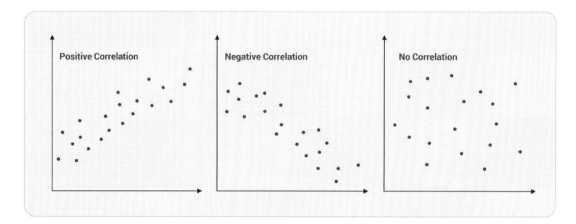

As shown in the figures above, an X-Y diagram may result in positive, negative, or no correlation between the two variables. So in the first scatter plot as the Y factor increases the X factor increases as well. The opposite is true as well: as the X factor increases the Y factor also increases. Thus there is a positive correlation because one factor appears to positively affect the other factor

It's important to note, however, that a positive correlation between two variables doesn't equate to a cause-and-effect relationship. For example, a positive correlation between labor hours and units produced may not equate to a cause and effect relationship between the two. Any instance of correlation only indicates how likely the presence of one variable is in the instance of another. The variables should be further analyzed to determine which, if any, other variables (i.e. quality of employee work) may contribute to the positive correlation.

<u>Comparing Data</u>

Comparing data sets within statistics can mean many things. The first way to compare data sets is by looking at the center and spread of each set. The center of a data set can mean two things: median or mean. The *median* is the value that's halfway into each data set, and it splits the data into two intervals. The *mean* is the average value of the data within a set. It's calculated by adding up all of the data in the set and dividing the total by the number of data points. Outliers can significantly impact the mean. Additionally, two completely different data sets can have the same mean. For example, a data set with values ranging from 0 to 100 and a data set with values ranging from 44 to 56 can both have means of 50. The first data set has a much wider range, which is known as the *spread* of the data. This measures how varied the data is within each set.

Explaining the Relationship between Two Variables

In an experiment, variables are the key to analyzing data, especially when data is in a graph or table. Variables can represent anything, including objects, conditions, events, and amounts of time.

Covariance is a general term referring to how two variables move in relation to each other. Take for example an employee that gets paid by the hour. For them, hours worked and total pay have a positive covariance. As hours worked increases, so does pay.

Constant variables remain unchanged by the scientist across all trials. Because they are held constant for all groups in an experiment, they aren't being measured in the experiment, and they are usually ignored. Constants can either be controlled by the scientist directly like the nutrition, water, and sunlight given to plants, or they can be selected by the scientist specifically for an experiment like using a certain animal species or choosing to investigate only people of a certain age group.

Independent variables are also controlled by the scientist, but they are the same only for each group or trial in the experiment. Each group might be composed of students that all have the same color of car or each trial may be run on different soda brands. The independent variable of an experiment is what is being indirectly tested because it effects change in the dependent variables.

Dependent variables experience change caused by the independent variable and are what is being measured or observed. For example, college acceptance rates could be a dependent variable of an experiment that sorted a large sample of high school students by an independent variable such as test scores. In this experiment, the scientist groups the high school students by the independent variable (test scores) to see how it affects the dependent variable (their college acceptance rates).

Note that most variables can be held constant in one experiment but independent or dependent in another. For example, when testing how well a fertilizer aids plant growth, its amount of sunlight should be held constant for each group of plants, but if the experiment is being done to determine the proper amount of sunlight a plant should have, the amount of sunlight is an independent variable because it is necessarily changed for each group of plants.

Calculating Geometric Quantities

Perimeter and Area
Perimeter is the measurement of a distance around something or the sum of all sides of a polygon. Think of perimeter as the length of the boundary, like a fence. In contrast, *area* is the space occupied by a defined enclosure, like a field enclosed by a fence.

When thinking about perimeter, think about walking around the outside of something. When thinking about area, think about the amount of space or *surface area* something takes up.

Square
The perimeter of a square is measured by adding together all of the sides. Since a square has four equal sides, its perimeter can be calculated by multiplying the length of one side by 4. Thus, the formula is $P = 4 \times s$, where s equals one side. For example, the following square has side lengths of 5 meters:

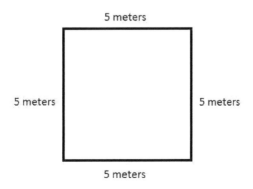

The perimeter is 20 meters because 4 times 5 is 20.

The area of a square is the length of a side squared, and the area of a rectangle is length multiplied by the width. For example, if the length of the square is 7 centimeters, then the area is 49 square centimeters. The formula for this example is $A = s^2 = 7^2 = 49$ square centimeters. An example of a rectangle is if the rectangle has a length of 6 inches and a width of 7 inches, then the area is 42 square inches:

$$A = lw = 6(7) = 42 \text{ square inches}$$

Rectangle
Like a square, a rectangle's perimeter is measured by adding together all of the sides. But as the sides are unequal, the formula is different. A rectangle has equal values for its lengths (long sides) and equal values for its widths (short sides), so the perimeter formula for a rectangle is:

$$P = l + l + w + w = 2l + 2w$$

l equals length
w equals width

The area is found by multiplying the length by the width, so the formula is $A = l \times w$.

For example, if the length of a rectangle is 10 inches and the width 8 inches, then the perimeter is 36 inches because:

$$P = 2l + 2w = 2(10) + 2(8) = 20 + 16 = 36 \text{ inches}$$

Triangle
A triangle's perimeter is measured by adding together the three sides, so the formula is $P = a + b + c$, where $a, b,$ and c are the values of the three sides. The area is the product of one-half the base and height so the formula is:

$$A = \frac{1}{2} \times b \times h$$

It can be simplified to:

$$A = \frac{bh}{2}$$

The base is the bottom of the triangle, and the height is the distance from the base to the peak. If a problem asks to calculate the area of a triangle, it will provide the base and height.

For example, if the base of the triangle is 2 feet and the height 4 feet, then the area is 4 square feet. The following equation shows the formula used to calculate the area of the triangle:

$$A = \frac{1}{2}bh = \frac{1}{2}(2)(4) = 4 \text{ square feet}$$

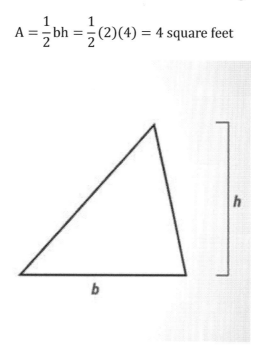

Circle

A circle's perimeter—also known as its circumference—is measured by multiplying the diameter by π.

Diameter is the straight line measured from one end to the direct opposite end of the circle.

π is referred to as pi and is equal to 3.14 (with rounding).

So the formula is $\pi \times d$.

This is sometimes expressed by the formula $C = 2 \times \pi \times r$, where r is the radius of the circle. These formulas are equivalent, as the radius equals half of the diameter.

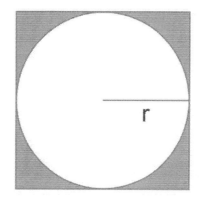

The area of a circle is calculated through the formula $A = \pi \times r^2$. The test will indicate either to leave the answer with π attached or to calculate to the nearest decimal place, which means multiplying by 3.14 for π.

Arc

The *arc of a circle* is the distance between two points on the circle. The length of the arc of a circle in terms of *degrees* is easily determined if the value of the central angle is known. The length of the arc is simply the value of the central angle. In this example, the length of the arc of the circle in degrees is 75°.

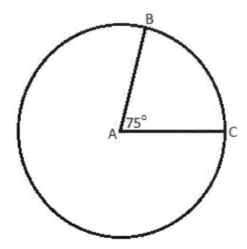

To determine the length of the arc of a circle in *distance*, the student will need to know the values for both the central angle and the radius. This formula is:

$$\frac{central\ angle}{360°} = \frac{arc\ length}{2\pi r}$$

The equation is simplified by cross-multiplying to solve for the arc length.

In the following example, the student should substitute the values of the central angle (75°) and the radius (10 inches) into the equation above to solve for the arc length.

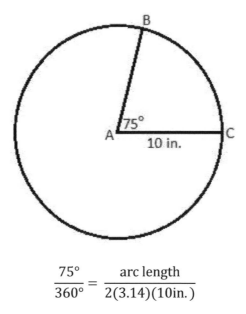

$$\frac{75°}{360°} = \frac{arc\ length}{2(3.14)(10in.)}$$

To solve the equation, first cross-multiply: 4710 = 360(arc length). Next, divide each side of the equation by 360. The result of the formula is that the arc length is 13.1 (rounded).

Irregular Shapes

The perimeter of an irregular polygon is found by adding the lengths of all of the sides. In cases where all of the sides are given, this will be very straightforward, as it will simply involve finding the sum of the provided lengths. Other times, a side length may be missing and must be determined before the perimeter can be calculated. Consider the example below:

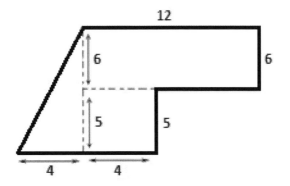

All of the side lengths are provided except for the angled side on the left. Test takers should notice that this is the hypotenuse of a right triangle. The other two sides of the triangle are provided (the base is 4 and the height is 6 + 5 = 11). The Pythagorean Theorem can be used to find the length of the hypotenuse, remembering that $a^2 + b^2 = c^2$.

Substituting the side values provided yields $(4)^2 + (11)^2 = c^2$.

Therefore, $c = \sqrt{16 + 121} = 11.7$

Finally, the perimeter can be found by adding this new side length with the other provided lengths to get the total length around the figure: 4 + 4 + 5 + 6 + 12 + 11.7 = 42.7. Although units are not provided in this figure, remember that reporting units with a measurement is important.

The area of an irregular polygon is found by decomposing, or breaking apart, the figure into smaller shapes. When the area of the smaller shapes is determined, these areas are added together to produce the total area of the area of the original figure. Consider the same example provided before:

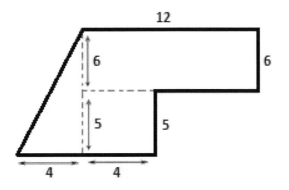

The irregular polygon is decomposed into two rectangles and a triangle. The area of the large rectangles $(A = l \times w \rightarrow A = 12 \times 6)$ is 72 square units. The area of the small rectangle is 20 square units $(A = 4 \times 5)$. The area of the triangle $(A = \frac{1}{2} \times b \times h \rightarrow A = \frac{1}{2} \times 4 \times 11)$ is 22 square units. The sum of the areas of these figures produces the total area of the original polygon: $A = 72 + 20 + 22 \rightarrow A = 114$ square units.

Converting Within and Between Standard and Metric Systems

<u>American Measuring System</u>
The measuring system used today in the United States developed from of the British units of measurement during colonial times. The most typically used units in this customary system are those used to measure weight, liquid volume, and length, whose common units are found below. In the customary system, the basic unit for measuring weight is the ounce (oz); there are 16 ounces (oz) in 1 pound (lb) and 2000 pounds in 1 ton. The basic unit for measuring liquid volume is the ounce (oz); 1 ounce is equal to 2 tablespoons (tbsp) or 6 teaspoons (tsp), and there are 8 ounces in 1 cup, 2 cups in 1 pint (pt), 2 pints in 1 quart (qt), and 4 quarts in 1 gallon (gal). For measurements of length, the inch (in) is the base unit; 12 inches make up 1 foot (ft), 3 feet make up 1 yard (yd), and 5280 feet make up 1 mile (mi). However, as there are only a set amount of units in the customary system, with extremely large or extremely small amounts of material, the numbers can become awkward and difficult to compare.

Common Customary Measurements		
Length	**Weight**	**Capacity**
1 foot = 12 inches	1 pound = 16 ounces	1 cup = 8 fluid ounces
1 yard = 3 feet	1 ton = 2,000 pounds	1 pint = 2 cups
1 yard = 36 inches		1 quart = 2 pints
1 mile = 1,760 yards		1 quart = 4 cups
1 mile = 5,280 feet		1 gallon = 4 quarts
		1 gallon = 16 cups

<u>Metric System</u>
Aside from the United States, most countries in the world have adopted the metric system embodied in the International System of Units (SI). The three main SI base units used in the metric system are the meter (m), the kilogram (kg), and the liter (L); meters measure length, kilograms measure mass, and liters measure volume.

These three units can use different prefixes, which indicate larger or smaller versions of the unit by powers of ten. This can be thought of as making a new unit which is sized by multiplying the original unit in size by a factor.

These prefixes and associated factors are:

Metric Prefixes			
Prefix	**Symbol**	**Multiplier**	**Exponential**
kilo	k	1,000	10^3
hecto	h	100	10^2
deca	da	10	10^1
no prefix		1	10^0
deci	d	0.1	10^{-1}
centi	c	0.01	10^{-2}
milli	m	0.001	10^{-3}

The correct prefix is then attached to the base. Some examples:

1 milliliter equals .001 liters.

1 kilogram equals 1,000 grams.

Choosing the Appropriate Measuring Unit

Some units of measure are represented as square or cubic units depending on the solution. For example, perimeter is measured in units, area is measured in square units, and volume is measured in cubic units.

Also be sure to use the most appropriate unit for the thing being measured. A building's height might be measured in feet or meters while the length of a nail might be measured in inches or centimeters. Additionally, for SI units, the prefix should be chosen to provide the most succinct available value. For example, the mass of a bag of fruit would likely be measured in kilograms rather than grams or milligrams, and the length of a bacteria cell would likely be measured in micrometers rather than centimeters or kilometers.

Conversion

Converting measurements in different units between the two systems can be difficult because they follow different rules. The best method is to look up an English to Metric system conversion factor and then use a series of equivalent fractions to set up an equation to convert the units of one of the measurements into those of the other. The table below lists some common conversion values that are useful for problems involving measurements with units in both systems:

English System	Metric System
1 inch	2.54 cm
1 foot	0.3048 m
1 yard	0.914 m
1 mile	1.609 km
1 ounce	28.35 g
1 pound	0.454 kg
1 fluid ounce	29.574 mL
1 quart	0.946 L
1 gallon	3.785 L

Consider the example where a scientist wants to convert 6.8 inches to centimeters. The table above is used to find that there are 2.54 centimeters in every inch, so the following equation should be set up and solved:

$$\frac{6.8\ in}{1} \times \frac{2.54\ cm}{1\ in} = 17.272\ cm$$

Notice how the inches in the numerator of the initial figure and the denominator of the conversion factor cancel out. (This equation could have been written simply as $6.8\ in \times 2.54\ cm = 17.272\ cm$, but it was shown in detail to illustrate the steps). The goal in any conversion equation is to set up the fractions so that the units you are trying to convert from cancel out and the units you desire remain.

For a more complicated example, consider converting 2.15 kilograms into ounces. The first step is to convert kilograms into grams and then grams into ounces. Note that the measurement you begin with does not have to be put in a fraction.

So in this case, 2.15 kg is by itself although it's technically the numerator of a fraction:

$$2.15 \; kg \; \times \frac{1000g}{kg} = 2150 \; g$$

Then, use the conversion factor from the table to convert grams to ounces:

$$2150g \; \times \frac{1 \; oz}{28.35g} = 75.8 \; oz$$

Practice Questions

1. Which of the following numbers has the greatest value?
    a. 1.4378
    b. 1.07548
    c. 1.43592
    d. 0.89409

2. The value of 6 x 12 is the same as:
    a. 2 x 4 x 4 x 2
    b. 7 x 4 x 3
    c. 6 x 6 x 3
    d. 3 x 3 x 4 x 2

3. This chart indicates how many sales of CDs, vinyl records, and MP3 downloads occurred over the last year. Approximately what percentage of the total sales was from CDs?

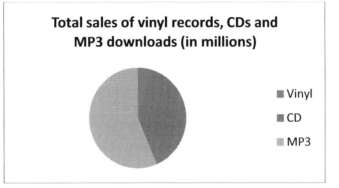

    a. 55%
    b. 25%
    c. 40%
    d. 5%

4. After a 20% sale discount, Frank purchased a new refrigerator for $850. How much did he save from the original price?
    a. $170
    b. $212.50
    c. $105.75
    d. $200

5. Which of the following is largest?
    a. 0.45
    b. 0.096
    c. 0.3
    d. 0.313

6. What is the value of *b* in this equation?

$$5b - 4 = 2b + 17$$

    a. 13
    b. 24
    c. 7
    d. 21

7. A school has 15 teachers and 20 teaching assistants. They have 200 students. What is the ratio of faculty to students?
    a. 3:20
    b. 4:17
    c. 3:2
    d. 7:40

8. Express the solution to the following problem in decimal form:

$$\frac{3}{5} \times \frac{7}{10} \div \frac{1}{2}$$

    a. 0.042
    b. 84%
    c. 0.84
    d. 0.42

9. A student gets an 85% on a test with 20 questions. How many answers did the student solve correctly?
    a. 15
    b. 16
    c. 17
    d. 18

10. If Sarah reads at an average rate of 21 pages in four nights, how long will it take her to read 140 pages?
    a. 6 nights
    b. 26 nights
    c. 8 nights
    d. 27 nights

11. Alan currently weighs 200 pounds, but he wants to lose weight to get down to 175 pounds. What is this difference in kilograms? (1 pound is approximately equal to 0.45 kilograms.)
    a. 9 kg
    b. 11.25 kg
    c. 78.75 kg
    d. 90 kg

12. Johnny earns $2334.50 from his job each month. He pays $1437 for monthly expenses. Johnny is planning a vacation in 3 months' time that he estimates will cost $1750 total. How much will Johnny have left over from three months' of saving once he pays for his vacation?
    a. $948.50
    b. $584.50
    c. $852.50
    d. $942.50

13. What is $\frac{420}{98}$ rounded to the nearest integer?
   a. 3
   b. 4
   c. 5
   d. 6

14. Solve the following:

$$4 \times 7 + (25 - 21)^2 \div 2$$

   a. 512
   b. 36
   c. 60.5
   d. 22

15. The total perimeter of a rectangle is 36 cm. If the length of each side is 12 cm, what is the width?
   a. 3 cm
   b. 12 cm
   c. 6 cm
   d. 8 cm

16. Dwayne has received the following scores on his math tests: 78, 92, 83, 97. What score must Dwayne get on his next math test to have an overall average of at least 90?
   a. 89
   b. 98
   c. 95
   d. 100

17. What is the overall median of Dwayne's current scores: 78, 92, 83, 97?
   a. 19
   b. 85
   c. 83
   d. 87.5

18. Solve the following:

$$\left(\sqrt{36} \times \sqrt{16}\right) - 3^2$$

   a. 30
   b. 21
   c. 15
   d. 13

19. In Jim's school, there are 3 girls for every 2 boys. There are 650 students in total. Using this information, how many students are girls?
   a. 260
   b. 130
   c. 65
   d. 390

20. What is the solution to 4 x 7 + (25 − 21)² ÷ 2?
    a. 512
    b. 36
    c. 60.5
    d. 22

21. Kimberley earns $10 an hour babysitting, and after 10 p.m., she earns $12 an hour, with the amount paid being rounded to the nearest hour accordingly. On her last job, she worked from 5:30 p.m. to 11 p.m. In total, how much did Kimberley earn on her last job?
    a. $45
    b. $57
    c. $62
    d. $42

22. Solve this equation:

$$9x + x − 7 = 16 + 2x$$

    a. -4

    b. 3

    c. $\frac{9}{8}$

    d. $\frac{23}{8}$

23. Arrange the following numbers from least to greatest value:
    $0.85, \frac{4}{5}, \frac{2}{3}, \frac{91}{100}$

    a. $0.85, \frac{4}{5}, \frac{2}{3}, \frac{91}{100}$

    b. $\frac{4}{5}, 0.85, \frac{91}{100}, \frac{2}{3}$

    c. $\frac{2}{3}, \frac{4}{5}, 0.85, \frac{91}{100}$

    d. $0.85, \frac{91}{100}, \frac{4}{5}, \frac{2}{3}$

24. Keith's bakery had 252 customers go through its doors last week. This week, that number increased to 378. Express this increase as a percentage.
    a. 26%
    b. 50%
    c. 35%
    d. 12%

25. If $4x − 3 = 5$, then $x =$
    a. 1
    b. 2
    c. 3
    d. 4

26. Simplify the following fraction:

$$\frac{\frac{5}{7}}{\frac{9}{11}}$$

a. $\frac{55}{63}$

b. $\frac{7}{1000}$

c. $\frac{13}{15}$

d. $\frac{5}{11}$

27. The following graph compares the various test scores of the top three students in each of these teacher's classes. Based on the graph, which teacher's students had the lowest range of test scores?

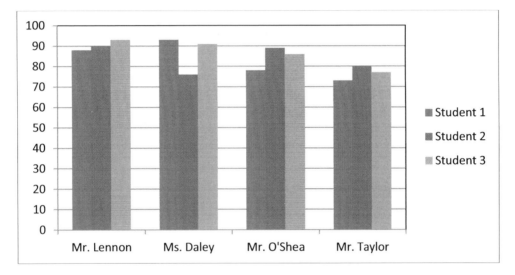

a. Mr. Lennon
b. Mr. O'Shea
c. Mr. Taylor
d. Ms. Daley

28. Bernard can make $80 per day. If he needs to make $300 and only works full days, how many days will this take?

a. 2
b. 3
c. 4
d. 5

29. Using the following diagram, calculate the total circumference, rounding to the nearest decimal place:

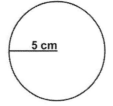

5 cm

    a. 25.0 cm
    b. 15.7 cm
    c. 78.5 cm
    d. 31.4 cm

30. Which measure for the center of a small sample set would be most affected by outliers?
    a. Mean
    b. Median
    c. Mode
    d. None of the above

31. A line that travels from the bottom-left of a graph to the upper-right of the graph indicates what kind of relationship between a predictor and a dependent variable?
    a. Positive
    b. Negative
    c. Exponential
    d. Logarithmic

32. How many kilometers is 4382 feet?
    a. 1.336 kilometers
    b. 14,376 kilometers
    c. 1.437 kilometers
    d. 13,336 kilometers

33. Which of the following is the best description of the relationship between Y and X?
    a. The data has normal distribution.
    b. X and Y have a negative relationship.
    c. No relationship
    d. X and Y have a positive relationship.

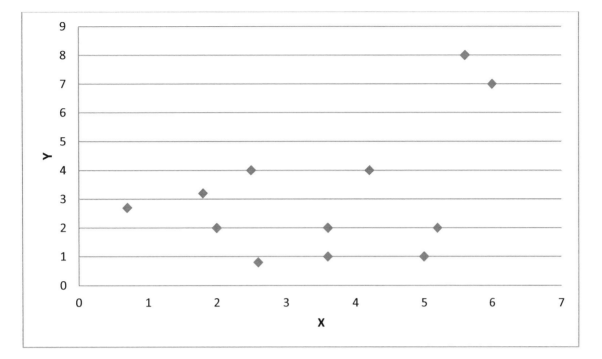

34. What is the slope of this line?

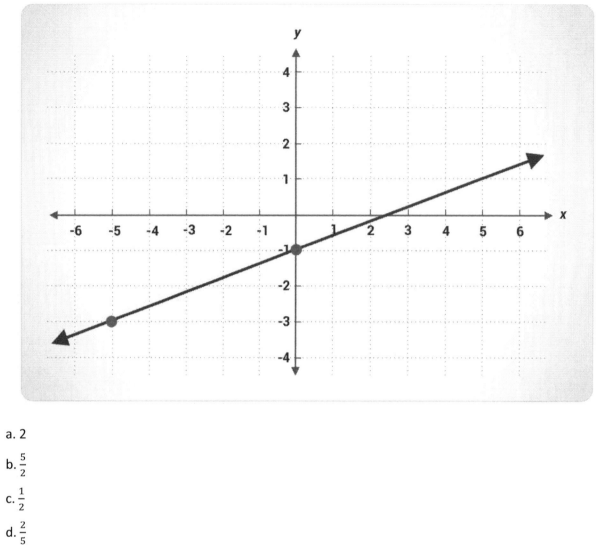

a. 2

b. $\frac{5}{2}$

c. $\frac{1}{2}$

d. $\frac{2}{5}$

35. What is the perimeter of the figure below? Note that the solid outer line is the perimeter.

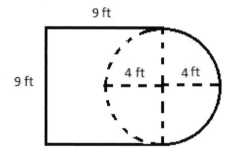

a. 48.565 ft
b. 39.565 ft
c. 19.78 ft
d. 30.565 ft

36. Which of the following equations best represents the problem below?

The width of a rectangle is 2 centimeters less than the length. If the perimeter of the rectangle is 44 centimeters, then what are the dimensions of the rectangle?

    a. $2l + 2(l - 2) = 44$
    b. $l + 2) + (l + 2) + l = 48$
    c. $l \times (l - 2) = 44$
    d. $(l + 2) + (l + 2) + l = 44$

Answer Explanations

1. A: Compare each numeral after the decimal point to figure out which overall number is greatest. In answers *A* (1.43785) and *C* (1.43592), both have the same tenths (4) and hundredths (3). However, the thousandths is greater in answer *A* (7), so *A* has the greatest value overall.

2. D: By grouping the four numbers in the answer into factors of the two numbers of the question (6 and 12), it can be determined that (3 x 2) x (4 x 3) = 6 x 12. Alternatively, each of the answer choices could be prime factored or multiplied out and compared to the original value. 6×12 has a value of 72 and a prime factorization of $2^3 \times 3^2$. The answer choices respectively have values of 64, 84, 108, and 72 and prime factorizations of 2^6, $2^2 \times 3 \times 7$, $2^2 \times 3^3$, and $2^3 \times 3^2$, so answer *D* is the correct choice.

3. C: The sum total percentage of a pie chart must equal 100%. Since the CD sales take up less than half of the chart and more than a quarter (25%), it can be determined to be 40% overall. This can also be measured with a protractor. The angle of a circle is 360°. Since 25% of 360 would be 90° and 50% would be 180°, the angle percentage of CD sales falls in between; therefore, it would be answer *C*.

4. B: Since $850 is the price *after* a 20% discount, $850 represents 80% of the original price. To determine the original price, set up a proportion with the ratio of the sale price (850) to original price (unknown) equal to the ratio of sale percentage:

$$\frac{850}{x} = \frac{80}{100}$$

(where *x* represents the unknown original price)

To solve a proportion, cross multiply the numerators and denominators and set the products equal to each other: (850)(100) = (80)(x). Multiplying each side results in the equation 85,000=80x.

To solve for *x*, divide both sides by 80: $\frac{85,000}{80} = \frac{80x}{80}$, resulting in x=1062.5. Remember that *x* represents the original price. Subtracting the sale price from the original price ($1062.50-$850) indicates that Frank saved $212.50.

5. A: To figure out which is largest, look at the first non-zero digits. Answer *B*'s first nonzero digit is in the hundredths place. The other three all have nonzero digits in the tenths place, so it must be *A*, *C*, or *D*. Of these, *A* has the largest first nonzero digit.

6. C: To solve for the value of b, both sides of the equation need to be equalized.

Start by cancelling out the lower value of -4 by adding 4 to both sides:

$$5b - 4 = 2b + 17$$

$$5b - 4 + 4 = 2b + 17 + 4$$

$$5b = 2b + 21$$

The variable b is the same on each side, so subtract the lower 2b from each side:

$$5b = 2b + 21$$

$$5b - 2b = 2b + 21 - 2b$$

$$3b = 21$$

Then divide both sides by 3 to get the value of b:

$$3b = 21$$

$$\frac{3b}{3} = \frac{21}{3}$$

$$b = 7$$

7. D: The total faculty is 15 + 20 = 35. So the ratio is 35:200. Then, divide both of these numbers by 5, since 5 is a common factor to both, with a result of 7:40.

8. C: The first step in solving this problem is expressing the result in fraction form. Separate this problem first by solving the division operation of the last two fractions. When dividing one fraction by another, invert or flip the second fraction and then multiply the numerator and denominator.

$$\frac{7}{10} \times \frac{2}{1} = \frac{14}{10}$$

Next, multiply the first fraction with this value:

$$\frac{3}{5} \times \frac{14}{10} = \frac{42}{50}$$

Decimals are expressions of 1 or 100%, so multiply both the numerator and denominator by 2 to get the fraction as an expression of 100.

$$\frac{42}{50} \times \frac{2}{2} = \frac{84}{100}$$

In decimal form, this would be expressed as 0.84.

9. C: 85% of a number means that number should be multiplied by 0.85: $0.85 \times 20 = \frac{85}{100} \times \frac{20}{1}$, which can be simplified to $\frac{17}{20} \times \frac{20}{1} = 17$. The answer is C.

10. D: This problem can be solved by setting up a proportion involving the given information and the unknown value. The proportion is:

$$\frac{21\ pages}{4\ nights} = \frac{140\ pages}{x\ nights}$$

Solving the proportion by cross-multiplying, the equation becomes $21x = 4 * 140$, where $x = 26.67$. Since it is not an exact number of nights, the answer is rounded up to 27 nights. Twenty-six nights would not give Sarah enough time.

11. B: Using the conversion rate, multiply the projected weight loss of 25 lb by $0.45 \frac{kg}{lb}$ to get the amount in kilograms (11.25 kg).

12. D: First, subtract $1437 from $2334.50 to find Johnny's monthly savings; this equals $897.50. Then, multiply this amount by 3 to find out how much he will have (in three months) before he pays for his vacation: this equals $2692.50. Finally, subtract the cost of the vacation ($1750) from this amount to find how much Johnny will have left: $942.50.

13. B: Dividing by 98 can be approximated by dividing by 100, which would mean shifting the decimal point of the numerator to the left by 2. The result is 4.2 which rounds to 4.

14. B: To solve this correctly, keep in mind the order of operations with the mnemonic PEMDAS (Please Excuse My Dear Aunt Sally). This stands for Parentheses, Exponents, Multiplication, Division, Addition, Subtraction. Taking it step by step, solve the parentheses first:

$$4 \times 7 + (4)^2 \div 2$$

Then, apply the exponent:

$$4 \times 7 + 16 \div 2$$

Multiplication and division are both performed next:

$$28 + 8 = 36$$

15. C: The formula for the perimeter of a rectangle is P=2L+2W, where P is the perimeter, L is the length, and W is the width. The first step is to substitute all of the data into the formula:

$$36 = 2(12) + 2W$$

Simplify by multiplying 2x12:

$$36 = 24 + 2W$$

Simplifying this further by subtracting 24 on each side, which gives:

$$36-24 = 24-24+2W$$

$$12 = 2W$$

Divide by 2:

$$6 = W$$

The width is 6 cm. Remember to test this answer by substituting this value into the original formula: 36 = 2(12) + 2(6).

16. D: To find the average of a set of values, add the values together and then divide by the total number of values. In this case, include the unknown value of what Dwayne needs to score on his next test, in order to solve it.

$$\frac{78 + 92 + 83 + 97 + x}{5} = 90$$

Add the unknown value to the new average total, which is 5. Then multiply each side by 5 to simplify the equation, resulting in:

$$78 + 92 + 83 + 97 + x = 450$$

$$350 + x = 450$$

$$x = 100$$

Dwayne would need to get a perfect score of 100 in order to get an average of at least 90.

Test this answer by substituting back into the original formula.

$$\frac{78 + 92 + 83 + 97 + 100}{5} = 90$$

17. D: For an even number of total values, the *median* is calculated by finding the *mean* or average of the two middle values once all values have been arranged in ascending order from least to greatest. In this case, $(92 + 83) \div 2$ would equal the median 87.5, answer *D*.

18. C: Follow the *order of operations* in order to solve this problem. Solve the parentheses first, and then follow the remainder as usual.

$$(6 \times 4) - 9$$

This equals $24 - 9$ or 15, answer *C*.

19. D: Three girls for every two boys can be expressed as a ratio: 3:2. This can be visualized as splitting the school into 5 groups: 3 girl groups and 2 boy groups. The number of students which are in each group can be found by dividing the total number of students by 5:

650 divided by 5 equals 1 part, or 130 students per group

To find the total number of girls, multiply the number of students per group (130) by how the number of girl groups in the school (3). This equals 390, answer *D*.

20. B: To solve this correctly, keep in mind the order of operations with the mnemonic PEMDAS (Please Excuse My Dear Aunt Sally). This stands for Parentheses, Exponents, Multiplication, Division, Addition, Subtraction. Taking it step by step, solve the parentheses first:

$$4 \times 7 + (4)^2 \div 2$$

Then, apply the exponent:

$$4 \times 7 + 16 \div 2$$

Multiplication and division are both performed next:

$$28 + 8 = 36$$

21. C: Kimberley worked 4.5 hours at the rate of \$10/h and 1 hour at the rate of \$12/h. The problem states that her pay is rounded to the nearest hour, so the 4.5 hours would round up to 5 hours at the rate of \$10/h. (5h)(\$10/h)+(1h)(\$12/h)= \$50+\$12= \$62.

22. D:

$9x + x - 7 = 16 + 2x$	Combine $9x$ and x.
$10x - 7 = 16 + 2x$	
$10x - 7 + 7 = 16 + 2x + 7$	Add 7 to both sides to remove (-7).
$10x = 23 + 2x$	
$10x - 2x = 23 + 2x - 2x$	Subtract 2x from both sides to move it to the other side of the equation.
$8x = 23$	
$\dfrac{8x}{8} = \dfrac{23}{8}$	Divide by 8 to get x by itself.
$x = \dfrac{23}{8}$	

23. C: The first step is to depict each number using decimals. $\frac{91}{100}$ = 0.91

Multiplying both the numerator and denominator of $\frac{4}{5}$ by 20 makes it $\frac{80}{100}$ or 0.80; the closest approximation of $\frac{2}{3}$ would be $\frac{66}{100}$ or 0.66 recurring. Rearrange each expression in ascending order, as found in answer C.

24. B: First, calculate the difference between the larger value and the smaller value.

$378 - 252 = 126$

To calculate this difference as a percentage of the original value, and thus calculate the percentage *increase*, divide 126 by 252, then multiply by 100 to reach the percentage = 50%, answer B.

25. B: Add 3 to both sides to get $4x = 8$. Then divide both sides by 4 to get $x = 2$.

26. A: First simplify the larger fraction by separating it into two. When dividing one fraction by another, remember to *invert* the second fraction and multiply the two as follows:

$$\frac{5}{7} \times \frac{11}{9}$$

The resulting fraction $\frac{55}{63}$ cannot be simplified further, so this is the answer to the problem.

27. A: To calculate the range in a set of data, subtract the highest value with the lowest value. In this graph, the range of Mr. Lennon's students is 5, which can be seen physically in the graph as having the smallest difference compared with the other teachers between the highest value and the lowest value.

28. C: 300/80 =30/8 = 15/4 =3.75. But Bernard is only working full days, so he will need to work 4 days, since 3 days is not sufficient.

29. D: To calculate the circumference of a circle, use the formula $2\pi r$, where r equals the radius or half of the diameter of the circle and $\pi = 3.14 \dots$. Substitute the given information, $2\pi 5 = 31.4 \dots$, answer D.

30. A: Mean. An outlier is a data value that's either far above or below the majority of values in a sample set. The mean is the average of all values in the set. In a small sample, a very high or low number could greatly change the average. The median is the middle value when arranged from lowest to highest. Outliers would have no more of an effect on the median than any other value. Mode is the value that repeats most often in a set. Assuming that the same outlier doesn't repeat, outliers would have no effect on the mode of a sample set.

31. A: This vector indicates a positive relationship. A negative relationship would show points traveling from the top-left of the graph to the bottom-right. Exponential and logarithmic functions aren't linear (don't create a straight line), so these options could have been immediately eliminated.

32. A: The conversion can be obtained by setting up and solving the following equation:

$$4382\ ft\ \times \frac{.3048\ m}{1\ ft} \times \frac{1\ km}{1000\ m} = 1.336\ km$$

33. C: There is no verifiable relationship between the two variables. While it may seem to have somewhat of a positive correlation because of the last two data points: (5.6,8) and (6,7), you must also take into account the two data points before those (5,1) and (5.2, 2) that have low Y values despite high X values. Data with a normal distribution (Choice A) has an arc to it. This data does not.

34. D: The slope is given by the change in *y* divided by the change in *x*. Specifically, it's:

$$slope = \frac{y_2 - y_1}{x_2 - x_1}$$

The first point is (-5,-3) and the second point is (0,-1). Work from left to right when identifying coordinates. Thus the point on the left is point 1 (-5,-3) and the point on the right is point 2 (0,-1).

Now we need to just plug those numbers into the equation:

$$slope = \frac{-1 - (-3)}{0 - (-5)}$$

It can be simplified to:

$$slope = \frac{-1 + 3}{0 + 5}$$

$$slope = \frac{2}{5}$$

35. B: The figure is composed of three sides of a square and a semicircle. The sides of the square are simply added: 9 + 9 + 9 = 27 feet. The circumference of a circle is found by the equation C = 2πr. The radius is 4, so the circumference of the circle is 25.13 ft. Only half of the circle makes up the outer border of the figure (part of the perimeter) so half of 25.13 feet is 12.565 ft. Therefore, the total perimeter is: 27 ft + 12.565 ft = 39.565 ft. The other answer choices use the incorrect formula or fail to include all of the necessary sides.

36. A: The first step is to determine the unknown, which is in terms of the length, l.

The second step is to translate the problem into the equation using the perimeter of a rectangle, $P = 2l + 2w$. The width is the length minus 2 centimeters. The resulting equation is $2l + 2(l - 2) = 44$. The equation can be solved as follows:

$2l + 2l - 4 = 44$	Apply the distributive property on the left side of the equation
$4l - 4 = 44$	Combine like terms on the left side of the equation
$4l = 48$	Add 4 to both sides of the equation
$l = 12$	Divide both sides of the equation by 4

The length of the rectangle is 12 centimeters. The width is the length minus 2 centimeters, which is 10 centimeters. Checking the answers for length and width forms the following equation:

$$44 = 2(12) + 2(10)$$

The equation can be solved using the order of operations to form a true statement: $44 = 44$.

Science

Human Anatomy and Physiology

General Anatomy and Physiology of a Human

Anatomy may be defined as the structural makeup of an organism. The study of anatomy may be divided into microscopic/fine anatomy and macroscopic/gross anatomy. Fine anatomy concerns itself with viewing the features of the body with the aid of a microscope, while gross anatomy concerns itself with viewing the features of the body with the naked eye. *Physiology* refers to the functions of an organism and it examines the chemical or physical functions that help the body function appropriately.

Levels of Organization of the Human Body
All the parts of the human body are built of individual units called *cells*. Groups of similar cells are arranged into *tissues,* different tissues are arranged into *organs,* and organs working together form entire *organ systems.* The human body has twelve organ systems that govern circulation, digestion, immunity, hormones, movement, support, coordination, urination & excretion, reproduction (male and female), respiration, and general protection.

Here are some of the systems of the body:

HUMAN BODY SYSTEMS

Circulatory System | Central nervous System | Respiratory System | Digestive System | Skeletal System | Muscular System

<u>Body Cavities</u>
The body is partitioned into different hollow spaces that house organs. The human body contains the following cavities:

- Cranial cavity: The cranial cavity is surrounded by the skull and contains organs such as the brain and pituitary gland.

- Thoracic cavity: The thoracic cavity is encircled by the sternum (breastbone) and ribs. It contains organs such as the lungs, heart, trachea (windpipe), esophagus, and bronchial tubes.

- Abdominal cavity: The abdominal cavity is separated from the thoracic cavity by the diaphragm. It contains organs such as the stomach, gallbladder, liver, small intestines, and large intestines. The abdominal organs are held in place by a membrane called the peritoneum.

- Pelvic cavity: The pelvic cavity is enclosed by the pelvis, or bones of the hip. It contains organs such as the urinary bladder, urethra, ureters, anus, and rectum. In females, the pelvic cavity also contains the uterus.

- Spinal cavity: The spinal cavity is surrounded by the vertebral column. The vertebral column has five regions: cervical, thoracic, lumbar, sacral, and coccygeal. The spinal cord runs through the middle of the spinal cavity.

<u>Human Tissues</u>
Human tissues can be grouped into four categories:

Muscle: Muscle tissue supports the body and allows it to move, and muscles are special as their cells have the ability to contract. There are three distinct types of muscle tissue: skeletal, smooth, and cardiac. Skeletal muscle is voluntary, or under conscious control, and is usually attached to bones. Most body movement is directly caused by the contraction of skeletal muscle. Smooth muscle is typically involuntary, or not under conscious control, and may be found in blood vessels, the walls of hollow organs, and the urinary bladder. Cardiac muscle is involuntary and found in the heart, which helps propel blood throughout the body.

Nervous: Nervous tissue is unique in that it is able to coordinate information from sensory organs as well as communicate the proper behavioral responses. Neurons, or nerve cells, are the workhorses of the nervous system. They communicate via action potentials (electrical signals) and neurotransmitters (chemical signals).

Epithelial: Epithelial tissue covers the external surfaces of organs and lines many of the body's cavities. Epithelial tissue helps to protect the body from invasion by microbes (bacteria, viruses, parasites), fluid loss, and injury.

Epithelial cell shapes can be:

- Squamous: cells with a flat shape
- Cuboidal: cells with a cubed shape
- Columnar: cells shaped like a column

Epithelial cells can be arranged in four patterns:

- Simple: a type of epithelium composed solely from a single layer of cells
- Stratified: a type of epithelium composed of multiple layers of cells

- Pseudostratified: a type of epithelium which appears to be stratified but in reality consists of only one layer of cells
- Transitional: a type of epithelium noted for its ability to expand and contract

Connective: Connective tissue supports and connects the tissues and organs of the body. Connective tissue is composed of cells dispersed throughout a matrix which can be gel, liquid, protein fibers, or salts. The primary protein fibers in the matrix are collagen (for strength), elastin (for flexibility), and reticulum (for support). Connective tissue can be categorized as either *loose* or *dense*. Examples of connective tissue include bones, cartilage, ligaments, tendons, blood, and adipose (fat) tissue.

Three Primary Body Planes

A plane is an imaginary flat surface. The three primary planes of the human body are frontal, sagittal, and transverse. The frontal, or coronal, plane is a vertical plane that divides the body or organ into front (anterior) and back (posterior) portions. The sagittal, or lateral, plane is a vertical plane divides the body or organ into right and left sides. The transverse, or axial, plane is a horizontal plane that divides the body or organ into upper and lower portions. In medical imaging, computed tomography (CT) scans are oriented only in the transverse plane; while magnetic resonance imaging (MRI) scans may be oriented in any of the three planes.

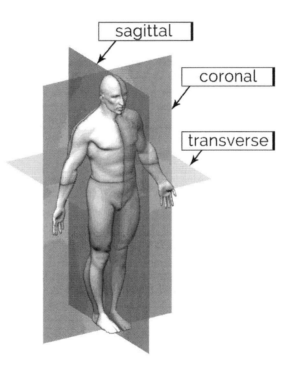

Terms of Direction

Medial refers to a structure being closer to the midline of the body. For example, the nose is medial to the eyes.

Lateral refers to a structure being farther from the midline of the body, and it is the opposite of *medial*. For example, the eyes are lateral to the nose.

Proximal refers to a structure or body part located near an attachment point. For example, the elbow is proximal to the wrist.

Distal refers to a structure or body part located far from an attachment point, and it is the opposite of *proximal*. For example, the wrist is distal to the elbow.

Anterior means toward the front in humans. For example, the lips are anterior to the teeth. The term *ventral* can be used in place of *anterior*.

Posterior means toward the back in humans, and it is the opposite of *anterior*. For example, the teeth are posterior to the lips. The term *dorsal* can be used in place of *posterior*.

Superior means above and refers to a structure closer to the head. For example, the head is superior to the neck. The terms *cephalic* or *cranial* may be used in place of *superior*.

Inferior means below and refers to a structure farther from the head, and it is the opposite of *superior*. For example, the neck is inferior to the head. The term *caudal* may be used in place of *inferior*.

Superficial refers to a structure closer to the surface. For example, the muscles are superficial because they are just beneath the surface of the skin.

Deep refers to a structure farther from the surface, and it is the opposite of *superficial*. For example, the femur is a deep structure lying beneath the muscles.

Body Regions
- Terms for general locations on the body include:
- Cervical: relating to the neck
- Clavicular: relating to the clavicle, or collarbone
- Ocular: relating to the eyes
- Acromial: relating to the shoulder
- Cubital: relating to the elbow
- Brachial: relating to the arm
- Carpal: relating to the wrist
- Thoracic : relating to the chest
- Abdominal: relating to the abdomen
- Pubic: relating to the groin
- Pelvic: relating to the pelvis, or bones of the hip
- Femoral: relating to the femur, or thigh bone
- Geniculate: relating to the knee
- Pedal: relating to the foot
- Palmar: relating to the palm of the hand
- Plantar: relating to the sole of the foot

Abdominopelvic Regions and Quadrants
The abdominopelvic region may be defined as the combination of the abdominal and the pelvic cavities. The region's upper border is the breasts and its lower border is the groin region. The region is divided into the following nine sections:

- Right hypochondriac: region below the cartilage of the ribs
- Epigastric: region above the stomach between the hypochondriac regions
- Left hypochondriac: region below the cartilage of the ribs
- Right lumbar: region of the waist
- Umbilical: region between the lumbar regions where the umbilicus, or belly button (navel), is located
- Left lumbar: region of the waist
- Right inguinal: region of the groin

- Hypogastric: region below the stomach between the inguinal regions
- Left inguinal: region of the groin

A simpler way to describe the abdominopelvic area would be to divide it into the following quadrants:

- Right upper quadrant (RUQ): Encompasses the right hypochondriac, right lumbar, epigastric, and umbilical regions.

- Right lower quadrant (RLQ): Encompasses the right lumbar, right inguinal, hypogastric, and umbilical regions.

- Left upper quadrant (LUQ): Encompasses the left hypochondriac, left lumbar, epigastric, and umbilical regions.

- Left lower quadrant (LLQ): Encompasses the left lumbar, left inguinal, hypogastric, and umbilical regions.

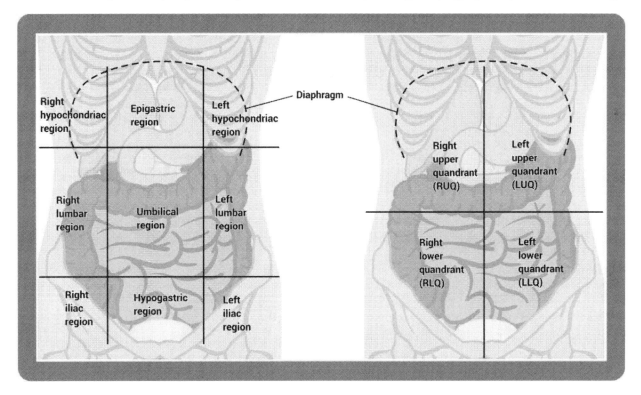

Cell Structure and Function
The cell is the main functional and structural component of all living organisms. Robert Hooke, an English scientist, coined the term "cell" in 1665. Hooke's discovery laid the groundwork for the cell theory, which is composed of three principals:

1. All organisms are composed of cells.

2. All existing cells are created from other living cells.

3. The cell is the most fundamental unit of life.

Organisms can be unicellular (composed of one cell) or multicellular (composed of many cells). All cells must be bounded by a cell membrane, be filled with cytoplasm of some sort, and be coded by a genetic sequence.

The cell membrane separates a cell's internal and external environments. It is a selectively permeable membrane, which usually only allows the passage of certain molecules by diffusion. Phospholipids and proteins are crucial components of all cell membranes. The cytoplasm is the cell's internal environment and is aqueous, or water-based. The genome represents the genetic material inside the cell that is passed on from generation to generation.

Prokaryotes and Eukaryotes

Prokaryotes are primitive organisms and have been around for billions of years. Eukaryotes evolved from prokaryotes and are much more complex organisms.

Prokaryotic cells are much smaller than eukaryotic cells. The majority of prokaryotes are unicellular, while the majority of eukaryotes are multicellular. Prokaryotic cells have no nucleus, and their genome is found in an area known as the nucleoid. They also do not have membrane-bound organelles, which are "little organs" that perform specific functions within a cell.

Eukaryotic cells have a proper nucleus containing the genome. They also have numerous membrane-bound organelles such as lysosomes, endoplasmic reticula (rough and smooth), Golgi complexes, and mitochondria. The majority of prokaryotic cells have cell walls, while most eukaryotic cells do not have cell walls. The DNA of prokaryotic cells is contained in a single circular chromosome, while the DNA of eukaryotic cells is contained in multiple linear chromosomes. Prokaryotic cells divide using binary fission, while eukaryotic cells divide using mitosis. Examples of prokaryotes are bacteria and archaea while examples of eukaryotes are animals and plants.

Nuclear Parts of a Cell

Nucleus (plural nuclei): Houses a cell's genetic material, deoxyribonucleic acid (DNA), which is used to form chromosomes. A single nucleus is the defining characteristic of eukaryotic cells. The nucleus of a cell controls gene expression. It ensures genetic material is transmitted from one generation to the next.

Chromosomes: Complex thread-like arrangements composed of DNA that is found in a cell's nucleus. Humans have 23 pairs of chromosomes for a total of 46.

Chromatin: An aggregate of genetic material consisting of DNA and proteins that forms chromosomes during cell division.

Nucleolus (plural nucleoli): The largest component of the nucleus of a eukaryotic cell. With no membrane, the primary function of the nucleolus is the production of ribosomes, which are crucial to the synthesis of proteins.

Cell Membranes

Cell membranes encircle the cell's cytoplasm, separating the intracellular environment from the extracellular environment. They are selectively permeable, which enables them to control molecular traffic entering and exiting cells. Cell membranes are made of a double layer of phospholipids studded with proteins. Cholesterol is also dispersed in the phospholipid bilayer of cell membranes to provide stability. The proteins in the phospholipid bilayer aid the transport of molecules across cell membranes.

Scientists use the term "fluid mosaic model" to refer to the arrangement of phospholipids and proteins in cell membranes. In that model, phospholipids have a head region and a tail region. The head region of the phospholipids is attracted to water (hydrophilic), while the tail region is repelled by it (hydrophobic). Because they are hydrophilic, the heads of the phospholipids are facing the water, pointing inside and outside of the cell. Because they are hydrophobic, the tails of the phospholipids are oriented inward between both head regions. This orientation constructs the phospholipid bilayer.

Cell membranes have the distinct trait of selective permeability. The fact that cell membranes are amphiphilic (having hydrophilic and hydrophobic zones) contributes to this trait. As a result, cell membranes are able to regulate the flow of molecules in and out of the cell.

Factors relating to molecules such as size, polarity, and solubility determine their likelihood of passage across cell membranes. Small molecules are able to diffuse easily across cell membranes compared to large molecules. Polarity refers to the charge present in a molecule. Polar molecules have regions, or poles, of positive and negative charge and are water soluble, while nonpolar molecules have no charge and are fat-soluble. Solubility refers to the ability of a substance, called a solute, to dissolve in a solvent. A soluble substance can be dissolved in a solvent, while an insoluble substance cannot be dissolved in a solvent. Nonpolar, fat-soluble substances have a much easier time passing through cell membranes compared to polar, water-soluble substances.

Passive Transport Mechanisms
Passive transport refers to the migration of molecules across a cell membrane that does not require energy. The three types of passive transport include simple diffusion, facilitated diffusion, and osmosis.

Simple diffusion relies on a concentration gradient, or differing quantities of molecules inside or outside of a cell. During simple diffusion, molecules move from an area of high concentration to an area of low concentration. Facilitated diffusion utilizes carrier proteins to transport molecules across a cell membrane. Osmosis refers to the transport of water across a selectively permeable membrane. During osmosis, water moves from a region of low solute concentration to a region of high solute concentration.

Active Transport Mechanisms
Active transport refers to the migration of molecules across a cell membrane that requires energy. It's a useful way to move molecules from an area of low concentration to an area of high concentration. Adenosine triphosphate (ATP), the currency of cellular energy, is needed to work against the concentration gradient.

Active transport can involve carrier proteins that cross the cell membrane to pump molecules and ions across the membrane, like in facilitated diffusion. The difference is that active transport uses the energy from ATP to drive this transport, as typically the ions or molecules are going against their concentration gradient. For example, glucose pumps in the kidney pump all of the glucose into the cells from the lumen of the nephron even though there is a higher concentration of glucose in the cell than in the lumen. This is because glucose is a precious food source and the body wants to conserve as much as possible. Pumps can either send a molecule in one direction, multiple molecules in the same direction (symports), or multiple molecules in different directions (antiports).

Active transport can also involve the movement of membrane-bound particles, either into a cell (endocytosis) or out of a cell (exocytosis). The three major forms of endocytosis are: pinocytosis, where the cell is *drinking* and intakes only small molecules; phagocytosis, where the cell is *eating* and intakes large particles or small organisms; and receptor-mediated endocytosis, where the cell's membrane splits off to form an internal vesicle as a response to molecules activating receptors on its surface. Exocytosis is the inverse of endocytosis, and the membranes of the vesicle join to that of the cell's surface while the molecules inside the vesicle are released outside. This is common in nervous and muscle tissue for the release of neurotransmitters and in endocrine cells for the release of hormones. The two major categories of exocytosis are excretion and secretion. Excretion is defined as the removal of waste from a cell. Secretion is defined as the transport of molecules from a cell such as hormones or enzymes.

Structure and Function of Cellular Organelles

Organelles are specialized structures that perform specific tasks in a cell. The term literally means "little organ." Most organelles are membrane bound and serve as sites for the production or degradation of chemicals. The following are organelles found in eukaryotic cells:

Nucleus: A cell's nucleus contains genetic information in the form of DNA. The nucleus is surrounded by the nuclear envelope. A single nucleus is the defining characteristic of eukaryotic cells. The nucleus is also the most important organelle of the cell. It contains the nucleolus, which manufactures ribosomes (another organelle) that are crucial in protein synthesis (also called gene expression).

Mitochondria: Mitochondria are oval-shaped and have a double membrane. The inner membrane has multiple folds called cristae. Mitochondria are responsible for the production of a cell's energy in the form of adenosine triphosphate (ATP). ATP is the principal energy transfer molecule in eukaryotic cells. Mitochondria also participate in cellular respiration.

Rough Endoplasmic Reticulum: The rough endoplasmic reticulum (RER) is composed of linked membranous sacs called cisternae with ribosomes attached to their external surfaces. The RER is responsible for the production of proteins that will eventually get shipped out of the cell.

Smooth Endoplasmic Reticulum: The smooth endoplasmic reticulum (SER) is composed of linked membranous sacs called cisternae without ribosomes, which distinguishes it from the RER. The SER's main function is the production of carbohydrates and lipids which can be created expressly for the cell or to modify the proteins from the RER that will eventually get shipped out of the cell.

Golgi Apparatus: The Golgi apparatus is located next to the SER. Its main function is the final modification, storage, and shipping of products (proteins, carbohydrates, and lipids) from the endoplasmic reticulum.

Lysosomes: Lysosomes are specialized vesicles that contain enzymes capable of digesting food, surplus organelles, and foreign invaders such as bacteria and viruses. They often destroy dead cells in order to recycle cellular components. Lysosomes are found only in animal cells.

Secretory Vesicles: Secretory vesicles transport and deliver molecules into or out of the cell via the cell membrane. Endocytosis refers to the movement of molecules into a cell via secretory vesicles. Exocytosis refers to the movement of molecules out of a cell via secretory vesicles.

Ribosomes: Ribosomes are not membrane bound. They are responsible for the production of proteins as specified from DNA instructions. Ribosomes can be free or bound.

Cilia and Flagella: Cilia are specialized hair-like projections on some eukaryotic cells that aid in movement, while flagella are long, whip-like projections that are used in the same capacity.

Here an illustration of the cell:

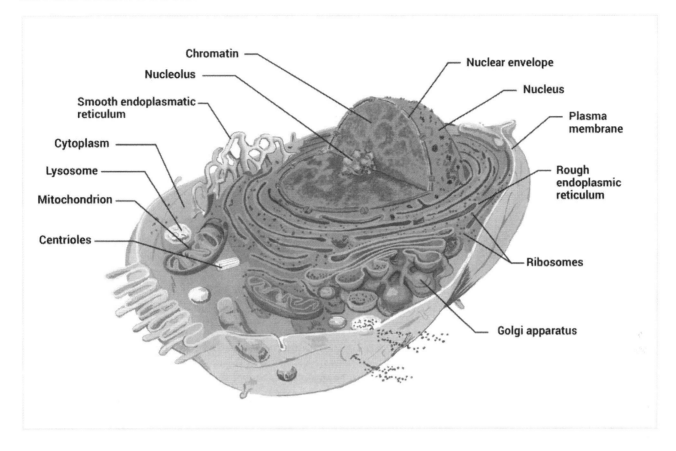

The following organelles are not found in animal cells:

Cell Walls: Cell walls can be found in plants, bacteria, and fungi, and are made of cellulose, peptidoglycan, and lignin according to the organism it is found around. Each of these materials is a type of sugar recognized as a structural carbohydrate. The carbohydrates are rigid structures located outside of the cell membrane. Cell walls function to protect the cell, help maintain a cell's shape, and provide structural support.

Vacuoles: Plant cells have central vacuoles, which are essentially a membrane surrounding a body of water. They may store nutrients or waste products. Since vacuoles are large, they also help to support the structure of plant cells.

Chloroplasts: Chloroplasts are membrane-bound organelles that perform photosynthesis. They contain structural units called thylakoids. Chlorophyll, a green pigment that circulates within the thylakoids, harnesses light energy (sunlight) and helps convert it into chemical energy (glucose).

Anatomy and Physiology of the Respiratory System

The respiratory system enables breathing and supports the energy-making process in our cells. The respiratory system transports an essential reactant, oxygen, to cells so that they can produce energy in their mitochondria via cellular respiration. The respiratory system also removes carbon dioxide, a waste product of cellular respiration.

This system is divided into the upper respiratory system and the lower respiratory system. The upper system comprises the nose, the nasal cavity and sinuses, and the pharynx. The lower respiratory system comprises the larynx (voice box), the trachea (windpipe), the small passageways leading to the lungs, and the lungs.

The pathway of oxygen to the bloodstream begins with the nose and the mouth. Upon inhalation, air enters the nose and mouth and passes into the sinuses where it gets warmed, filtered, and humidified. The throat, or the pharynx, allows the entry of both food and air; however, only air moves into the trachea, or windpipe, since the epiglottis covers the trachea during swallowing and prevents food from entering. The trachea contains mucus and cilia. The mucus traps many airborne pathogens while the cilia act as bristles that sweep the pathogens away toward the top of the trachea where they are either swallowed or coughed out.

The trachea itself has two vocal cords at the top which make up the larynx. At its bottom, the trachea forks into two major bronchi—one for each lung. These bronchi continue to branch into smaller and smaller bronchioles before terminating in grape-like air sacs called alveoli; these alveoli are surrounded by capillaries and provide the body with an enormous amount of surface area to exchange oxygen and carbon dioxide gases.

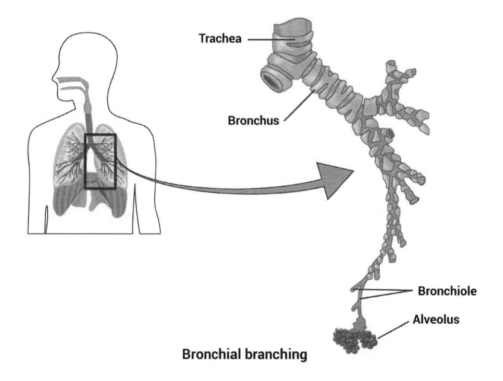

Bronchial branching

In total, the lungs contain about 1500 miles of airway passages. The right lung is divided into three lobes (superior, middle, and inferior), and the left lung is divided into two lobes (superior and inferior).

The left lung is smaller than the right lung, likely because it shares its space in the chest cavity with the heart.

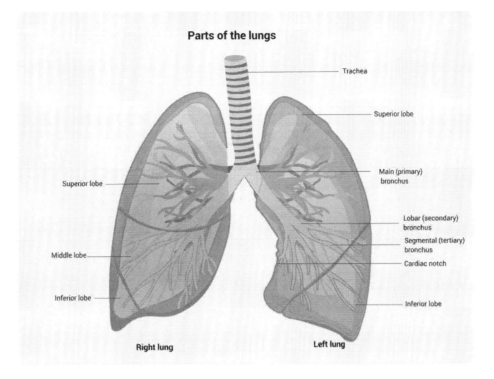

A flat muscle underneath the lungs called the diaphragm controls breathing. When the diaphragm contracts, the volume of the chest cavity increases and indirectly decreases its air pressure. This decrease in air pressure creates a vacuum, and the lungs pull in air to fill the space. This difference in air pressure that pulls the air from outside of the body into the lungs in a process called negative pressure breathing.

Upon inhalation or *inspiration*, oxygen in the alveoli diffuses into the capillaries to be carried by blood to cells throughout the body. A protein called hemoglobin in red blood cells easily bonds with oxygen, removing it from the blood and allowing more oxygen to diffuse in. This protein allows the blood to take in 60 times more oxygen than the body could without it, and this explains how oxygen can become so concentrated in blood even though it is only 21% of the atmosphere. While oxygen diffuses from the alveoli into the capillaries, carbon dioxide diffuses from the capillaries into the alveoli. When the diaphragm relaxes, the elastic lungs snap back to their original shape; this decreases the volume of the chest cavity and increases the air pressure until it is back to normal. This increased air pressure pushes the carbon dioxide waste from the alveoli through exhalation or *expiration*.

The autonomic nervous system controls breathing. The medulla oblongata gets feedback regarding the carbon dioxide levels in the blood, and will send a message to the diaphragm that it is time for a contraction. While breathing can be voluntary, it is mostly under autonomic control.

Functions of the Respiratory System
The respiratory system has many functions. Most importantly, it provides a large area for gas exchange between the air and the circulating blood. It protects the delicate respiratory surfaces from environmental variations and defends them against pathogens. It is responsible for producing the sounds that the body makes for speaking and singing, as well as for non-verbal communication. It also helps regulate blood volume and blood pressure by releasing vasopressin, and it is a regulator of blood pH due to its control over carbon dioxide release, as the aqueous form of carbon dioxide is the chief buffering agent in blood.

Anatomy and Physiology of the Cardiovascular System

The cardiovascular system (also called the circulatory system) is a network of organs and tubes that transport blood, hormones, nutrients, oxygen, and other gases to cells and tissues throughout the body. It is also known as the cardiovascular system. The major components of the circulatory system are the blood vessels, blood, and heart.

Blood Vessels
In the circulatory system, blood vessels are responsible for transporting blood throughout the body. The three major types of blood vessels in the circulatory system are arteries, veins, and capillaries. Arteries carry blood from the heart to the rest of the body. Veins carry blood from the body to the heart. Capillaries connect arteries to veins and form networks that exchange materials between the blood and the cells.

In general, arteries are stronger and thicker than veins as they need to withstand the high pressures exerted by the blood as the heart pumps it through the body. Arteries control blood flow through either vasoconstriction (narrowing of the blood vessel's diameter) or vasodilation (widening of the blood vessel's diameter). The blood in veins is under much lower pressures, so veins have valves to prevent the backflow of blood.

Most of the exchange between the blood and tissues takes place through the capillaries. There are three types of capillaries: continuous, fenestrated, and sinusoidal.

Continuous capillaries are made up of epithelial cells tightly connected together. As a result, they limit the types of materials that pass into and out of the blood. Continuous capillaries are the most common type of capillary. Fenestrated capillaries have openings that allow materials to be freely exchanged between the blood and tissues. They are commonly found in the digestive, endocrine, and urinary systems. Sinusoidal capillaries have larger openings and allow proteins and blood cells through. They are found primarily in the liver, bone marrow, and spleen.

Blood
Blood is vital to the human body. It is a liquid connective tissue that serves as a transport system for supplying cells with nutrients and carrying away their wastes. The average adult human has five to six quarts of blood circulating through their body. Approximately 55% of blood is plasma (the fluid portion), and the remaining 45% is composed of solid cells and cell parts. There are three major types of blood cells:

- Red blood cells transport oxygen throughout the body. They contain a protein called hemoglobin that allows them to carry oxygen. The iron in the hemoglobin gives the cells and the blood their red colors.

- White blood cells are responsible for fighting infectious diseases and maintaining the immune system. There are five types of white blood cells: neutrophils, lymphocytes, eosinophils, monocytes, and basophils.

- Platelets are cell fragments which play a central role in the blood clotting process.

All blood cells in adults are produced in the bone marrow—red blood cells from red marrow and white blood cells from yellow marrow.

Heart
The heart is a two-part, muscular pump that forcefully pushes blood throughout the human body. The human heart has four chambers—two upper atria and two lower ventricles, a pair on the left and a pair on the right. Anatomically, *left* and *right* correspond to the sides of the body that the patient themselves would refer to as left and right.

Four valves help to section off the chambers from one another. Between the right atrium and ventricle, the three flaps of the tricuspid valve keep blood from backflowing from the ventricle to the atrium, similar to how the two flaps of the mitral valve work between the left atrium and ventricle. As these two valves lie between an atrium and a ventricle, they are referred to as atrioventricular (AV) valves. The other two valves are semilunar (SL) and control blood flow into the two great arteries leaving the ventricles. The pulmonary valve connects the right ventricle to the pulmonary artery while the aortic valve connects the left ventricle to the aorta.

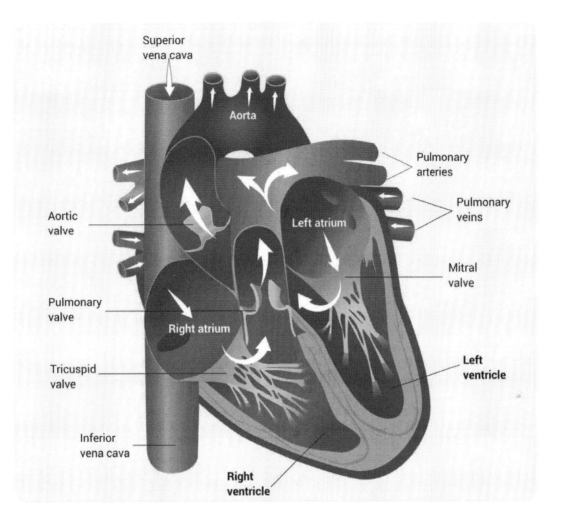

Cardiac Cycle
A cardiac cycle is one complete sequence of cardiac activity. The cardiac cycle represents the relaxation and contraction of the heart and can be divided into two phases: diastole and systole.

Diastole is the phase during which the heart relaxes and fills with blood. It gives rise to the diastolic blood pressure (DBP), which is the bottom number of a blood pressure reading. Systole is the phase during which the heart contracts and discharges blood. It gives rise to the systolic blood pressure (SBP), which is the top number of a blood pressure reading. The heart's electrical conduction system coordinates the cardiac cycle.

Types of Circulation
Five major blood vessels manage blood flow to and from the heart: the superior and inferior venae cavae, the aorta, the pulmonary artery, and the pulmonary vein.

The superior vena cava is a large vein that drains blood from the head and upper body. The inferior vena cava is a large vein that drains blood from the lower body. The aorta is the largest artery in the human body and carries blood from the heart to body tissues. The pulmonary arteries carry blood from the heart to the lungs. The pulmonary veins transport blood from the lungs to the heart.

In the human body, there are two types of circulation: pulmonary circulation and systemic circulation. Pulmonary circulation supplies blood to the lungs. Deoxygenated blood enters the right atrium of the heart and is routed through the tricuspid valve into the right ventricle. Deoxygenated blood then travels from the right ventricle of the heart through the pulmonary valve and into the pulmonary arteries. The pulmonary arteries carry the deoxygenated blood to the lungs. In the lungs, oxygen is absorbed and carbon dioxide is released. The pulmonary veins carry oxygenated blood to the left atrium of the heart.

Systemic circulation supplies blood to all other parts of the body, except the lungs. Oxygenated blood flows from the left atrium of the heart through the mitral, or bicuspid, valve into the left ventricle of the heart. Oxygenated blood is then routed from the left ventricle of the heart through the aortic valve and into the aorta. The aorta delivers blood to the systemic arteries, which supply the body tissues. In the tissues, oxygen and nutrients are exchanged for carbon dioxide and other wastes. The deoxygenated blood along with carbon dioxide and wastes enter the systemic veins, where they are returned to the right atrium of the heart via the superior and inferior vena cava.

Anatomy and Physiology of the Gastrointestinal System

The human body relies completely on the digestive system to meet its nutritional needs. After food and drink are ingested, the digestive system breaks them down into their component nutrients and absorbs them so that the circulatory system can transport them to other cells to use for growth, energy, and cell repair. These nutrients may be classified as proteins, lipids, carbohydrates, vitamins, and minerals.

The digestive system is thought of chiefly in two parts: the digestive tract (also called the alimentary tract or gastrointestinal tract) and the accessory digestive organs. The digestive tract is the pathway in which food is ingested, digested, absorbed, and excreted. It is composed of the mouth, pharynx, esophagus, stomach, small and large intestines, rectum, and anus. *Peristalsis*, or wave-like contractions of smooth muscle, moves food and wastes through the digestive tract. The accessory digestive organs are the salivary glands, liver, gallbladder, and pancreas.

Mouth and Stomach
The mouth is the entrance to the digestive system. Here, the mechanical and chemical digestion of the food begins. The food is chewed mechanically by the teeth and shaped into a *bolus* by the tongue so that it can be more easily swallowed by the esophagus. The food also becomes more watery and pliable with the addition of saliva secreted from the salivary glands, the largest of which are the parotid glands. The glands also secrete amylase in the saliva, an enzyme which begins chemical digestion and breakdown of the carbohydrates and sugars in the food.

The food then moves through the pharynx and down the muscular esophagus to the stomach.

The stomach is a large, muscular sac-like organ at the distal end of the esophagus. Here, the bolus is subjected to more mechanical and chemical digestion. As it passes through the stomach, it is physically squeezed and crushed while additional secretions turn it into a watery nutrient-filled liquid that exits into the small intestine as *chyme*.

The stomach secretes a great many substances into the *lumen* of the digestive tract. Some cells produce gastrin, a hormone that prompts other cells in the stomach to secrete a gastric acid composed mostly of hydrochloric acid (HCl). The HCl is at such a high concentration and low pH that it denatures most proteins and degrades a lot of organic matter. The stomach also secretes mucous to form a protective film that keeps the corrosive acid from dissolving its own cells. Gaps in this mucous layer can lead to peptic ulcers. Finally, the stomach also uses digestive enzymes like proteases and lipases to break down proteins and fats; although there are some gastric lipases here, the stomach is most known for breaking down proteins.

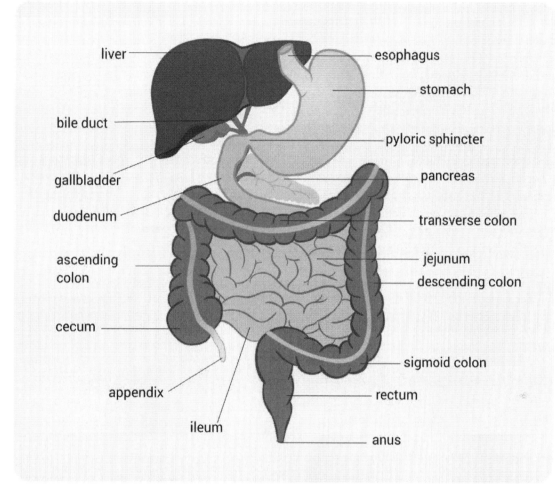

Small Intestine
The chyme from the stomach enters the first part of the small intestine, the *duodenum*, through the *pyloric sphincter*, and its extreme acidity is partly neutralized by sodium bicarbonate secreted along with mucous. The presence of chyme in the duodenum triggers the secretion of the hormones secretin and cholecystokinin (CCK). Secretin acts on the pancreas to dump more sodium bicarbonate into the small intestine so that the pH is kept at a reasonable level, while CCK acts on the gallbladder to release the *bile* that it has been storing. Bile is a substance produced by the liver and stored in the gallbladder which helps to *emulsify* or dissolve fats and lipids.

Because of the bile which aids in lipid absorption and the secreted lipases which break down fats, the duodenum is the chief site of fat digestion in the body. The duodenum also represents the last major site of chemical digestion in the digestive tract, as the other two sections of the small intestine (the *jejunum* and *ileum*) are instead heavily involved in absorption of nutrients.

The small intestine reaches 40 feet in length, and its cells are arranged in small finger-like projections called villi. This is due to its key role in the absorption of nearly all nutrients from the ingested and digested food, effectively transferring them from the lumen of the GI tract to the bloodstream where they travel to the cells which need them. These nutrients include simple sugars like glucose from carbohydrates, amino acids from proteins, emulsified fats, electrolytes like sodium and potassium, minerals like iron and zinc, and vitamins like D and B12. Vitamin B12's absorption, though it takes place in the intestines, is actually aided by *intrinsic factor* that was released into the chyme back in the stomach.

Large Intestine
The leftover parts of food which remain unabsorbed or undigested in the lumen of the small intestine next travel through the large intestine, which may also be referred to as the large bowel or colon. The large intestine is mainly responsible for water absorption. As the chyme at this stage no longer has anything useful that can be absorbed by the body, it is now referred to as *waste*, and it is stored in the large intestine until it can be excreted from the body. Removing the liquid from the waste transforms it from liquid to solid stool, or feces.

This waste first passes from the small intestine to the cecum, a pouch which forms the first part of the large intestine. In herbivores, it provides a place for bacteria to digest cellulose, but in humans most of it is vestigial and is known as the appendix. From the cecum, waste next travels up the ascending colon, across the transverse colon, down the descending colon, and through the sigmoid colon to the rectum. The rectum is responsible for the final storage of waste before being expelled through the . The anal canal is a small portion of the rectum leading through to the anus and the outside of the body.

Pancreas
The pancreas has endocrine and exocrine functions. The endocrine function involves releasing the hormones insulin, which decreases blood sugar (glucose) levels, and glucagon, which increases blood sugar (glucose) levels, directly into the bloodstream. Both hormones are produced in the islets of Langerhans, insulin in the beta cells and glucagon in the alpha cells.

The major part of the gland has exocrine function, which consists of acinar cells secreting inactive digestive enzymes (zymogens) into the main pancreatic duct. The main pancreatic duct joins the common bile duct, which empties into the small intestine (specifically the duodenum). The digestive enzymes are then activated and take part in the digestion of carbohydrates, proteins, and fats within chyme (the mixture of partially digested food and digestive juices).

Anatomy and Physiology of the Neuromuscular System

Nervous System
The human nervous system coordinates the body's response to stimuli from inside and outside the body. There are two major types of nervous system cells: neurons and neuroglia. Neurons are the workhorses of the nervous system and form a complex communication network that transmits electrical impulses termed action potentials, while neuroglia connect and support them.

Although some neurons monitor the senses, some control muscles, and some connect the brain to others, all neurons have four common characteristics:

- Dendrites: These receive electrical signals from other neurons across small gaps called *synapses*.
- Nerve cell body: This is the hub of processing and protein manufacture for the neuron.
- Axon: This transmits the signal from the cell body to other neurons.
- Terminals: These bridge the neuron to dendrites of other neurons and deliver the signal via chemical messengers called neurotransmitters.

Here an illustration of this:

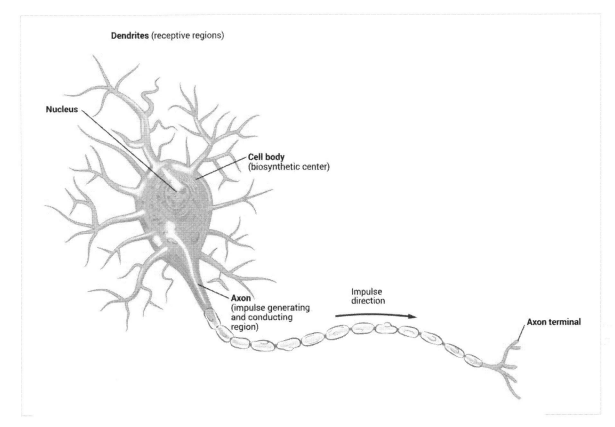

There are two major divisions of the nervous system: central and peripheral:

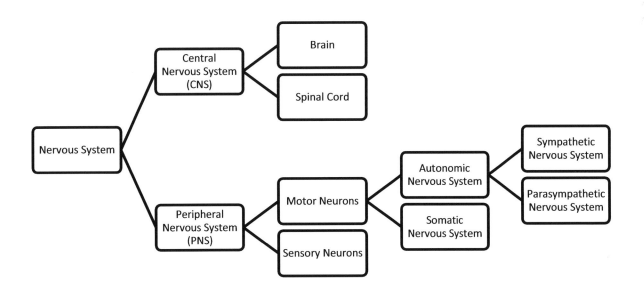

Central Nervous System

The central nervous system (CNS) consists of the brain and spinal cord. Three layers of membranes called the meninges cover and separate the CNS from the rest of the body.

The major divisions of the brain are the forebrain, the midbrain, and the hindbrain.

The forebrain consists of the cerebrum, the thalamus and hypothalamus, and the rest of the limbic system. The *cerebrum* is the largest part of the brain, and its most well-documented part is the outer cerebral cortex. The cerebrum is divided into right and left hemispheres, and each cerebral cortex hemisphere has four discrete areas, or lobes: frontal, temporal, parietal, and occipital. The frontal lobe governs duties such as voluntary movement, judgment, problem solving, and planning, while the other lobes are more sensory. The temporal lobe integrates hearing and language comprehension, the parietal lobe processes sensory input from the skin, and the occipital lobe functions to process visual input from the eyes. For completeness, the other two senses, smell and taste, are processed via the olfactory bulbs. The thalamus helps organize and coordinate all of this sensory input in a meaningful way for the brain to interpret.

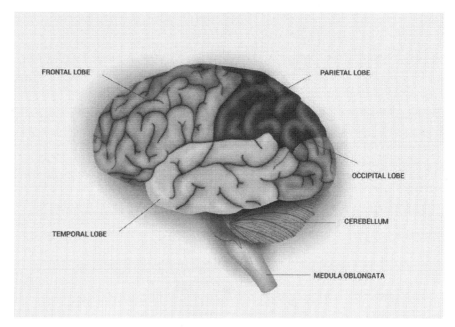

The hypothalamus controls the endocrine system and all of the hormones that govern long-term effects on the body. Each hemisphere of the limbic system includes a hippocampus (which plays a vital role in memory), an amygdala (which is involved with emotional responses like fear and anger), and other small bodies and nuclei associated with memory and pleasure.

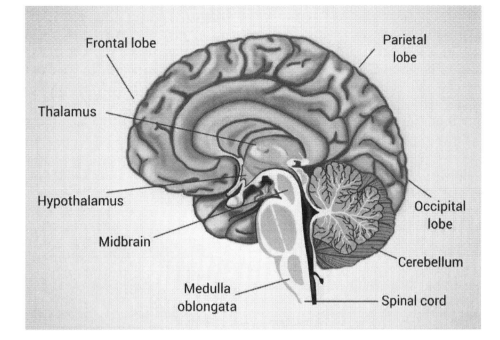

The midbrain is in charge of alertness, sleep/wake cycles, and temperature regulation, and it includes the substantia nigra which produces melatonin to regulate sleep patterns. The notable components of the hindbrain include the medulla oblongata and cerebellum. The medulla oblongata is located just above the spinal cord and is responsible for crucial involuntary functions such as breathing, heart rate, swallowing, and the regulation of blood pressure. Together with other parts of the hindbrain, the midbrain and medulla oblongata form the brain stem. The brain stem connects the spinal cord to the rest of the brain. To the rear of the brain stem sits the cerebellum which plays key roles in posture, balance, and muscular coordination. The spinal cord itself carries sensory information to the brain and motor information to the body, encapsulated by its protective bony spinal column.

Peripheral Nervous System
The peripheral nervous system (PNS) includes all nervous tissue besides the brain and spinal cord. The PNS consists of the sets of cranial and spinal nerves and relays information between the CNS and the rest of the body. The PNS has two divisions: the autonomic nervous system and the somatic nervous system.

Autonomic Nervous System
The autonomic nervous system (ANS) governs involuntary, or reflexive, body functions. Ultimately, the autonomic nervous system controls functions such as breathing, heart rate, digestion, body temperature, and blood pressure.

The ANS is split between parasympathetic nerves and sympathetic nerves. These two nerve types are antagonistic, and have opposite effects on the body. Parasympathetic nerves typically are useful when resting or during safe conditions and decrease heart rate, decrease inhalation speed, prepare digestion, and allow urination and excretion. Sympathetic nerves, on the other hand, become active when a person is under stress or excited, and they increase heart rate, increase breathing rates, and inhibit digestion, urination, and excretion.

Somatic Nervous System and the Reflex Arc
The somatic nervous system (SNS) governs the conscious, or voluntary, control of skeletal muscles and their corresponding body movements. The SNS contains afferent, or sensory, neurons and efferent, or motor, neurons. Afferent neurons carry sensory messages from the skeletal muscles, skin, or sensory organs to the CNS. Efferent neurons relay motor messages from the CNS to skeletal muscles, skin, or sensory organs.

The SNS also has a role in involuntary movements called reflexes. A reflex is defined as an involuntary response to a stimulus. They are transmitted via what is termed a *reflex arc*, where a stimulus is sensed by an affector and its afferent neuron, interpreted and rerouted by an interneuron, and delivered to effector muscles by an efferent neuron where they respond to the initial stimulus. A reflex is able to bypass the brain by being rerouted through the spinal cord; the interneuron decides the proper course of action rather than the brain. The reflex arc results in an instantaneous, involuntary response. For example, a physician tapping on the knee produces an involuntary knee jerk referred to as the patellar tendon reflex.

Muscular System
The muscular system is responsible for involuntary and voluntary movement of the body. There are three types of muscle: skeletal, cardiac, and smooth.

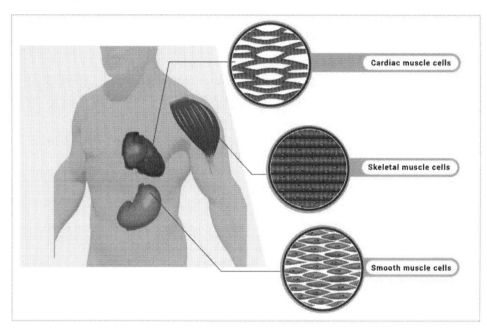

Skeletal Muscles
Skeletal muscles are attached to bones by tendons and are responsible for voluntary movement. The connecting tendons are made up of dense bands of connective tissue and have collagen fibers that firmly attach the muscle to the bone. Their fibers are actually woven into the coverings of the bone and muscle so that they can withstand pressure and tension. They usually work in opposing pairs like the bicep and tricep, for example.

Skeletal muscles are made of bundles of long fibers that are composed of cells with many nuclei due to their length. These fibers contain myofibrils, and myofibrils are made of alternating filaments. The thicker myosin filaments are in between the smaller actin filaments in a unit called a sarcomere, and the overlapping regions give the muscle their characteristic striated, or striped, appearance. Actin filaments are attached to exterior Z lines, myosin filaments are attached to a central M line, and when a muscle is at rest, there is a gap between the Z line and the myosin filaments. Only when the muscle contracts and the actin filaments slide over the myosin filaments does the myosin reach the Z line, as illustrated in the picture below. This sliding-filament model of

144

muscle contraction is dependent on myosin molecules forming and breaking cross-bridges with actin in order to pull the actin filaments closer to the M line.

Skeletal muscles are controlled by the nervous system. Motor neurons connect to muscle fibers via neuromuscular junctions. Motor neurons must release the neurotransmitter acetylcholine which releases calcium ions to stimulate myosin cross-bridging and contraction. As the acetylcholine stops being released, the contraction ends.

Smooth Muscles
Smooth muscles are responsible for involuntary movement like food moving through the digestive tract and blood moving through vessels. They have only one nucleus and do not have striations because actin and myosin filaments do not have an organized arrangement like skeletal muscles do. Unlike skeletal muscle, these muscles don't require neuromuscular junctions. Instead, they operate via gap junctions which send impulses directly from cell to cell.

Cardiac Muscles
Cardiac muscles are found only in the heart where they control the heart's rhythm and blood pressure. Like skeletal muscle, cardiac muscle has striations, but cardiac muscle cells are smaller than skeletal muscle cells, so they typically have only one nucleus. Like smooth muscle, cardiac muscles do not require neurotransmitter release by motor neurons to function, and they instead operate via gap junctions.

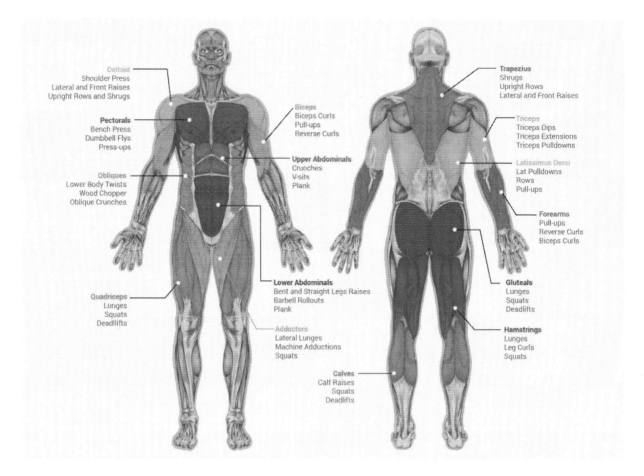

Anatomy and Physiology of the Reproductive System

The reproductive system is responsible for producing, storing, nourishing, and transporting functional reproductive cells, or gametes, in the human body. It includes the reproductive organs, also known as gonads, the reproductive tract, the accessory glands and organs that secrete fluids into the reproductive tract, and the perineal structures, which are the external genitalia.

Reproduction involves the passing of genes from one generation to the next, and that is accomplished through haploid gametes. Gametes have gone through meiosis and have 23 chromosomes, half the normal number. The male gamete is sperm, and the female gamete is an egg or ovum. When a sperm fertilizes an egg, they create a zygote which is the first cell of a new organism. The zygote has a full set of 46 chromosomes because it received 23 from each parent. Because of sperm and egg development gene shuffling, sperm and egg chromosome sets are all different which results in the variety seen in humans.

Male Reproductive System
The entire male reproductive system is designed to generate sperm and produce semen that facilitate fertilization of eggs, the female gametes. The testes are the endocrine glands that secrete testosterone, a

hormone that is important for secondary sex characteristics and sperm development, or spermatogenesis. Testosterone is in the androgen steroid-hormone family. The testes also produce and store 500 million spermatocytes, which are the male gametes, each day. Testes are housed in the scrotum which is a sac that hangs outside the body so that spermatogenesis occurs at cooler and optimal conditions.

The seminiferous tubules within the testes produce sperm and then they travel to epididymis where they are stored as they mature. Then, the sperm move to the ejaculatory duct via the vas deference. The ejaculatory duct contains more than just sperm. The seminal vesicles secrete an alkaline substance that will help sperm survive in the acidic vagina. The prostate gland secretes enzymes bathed in a milky white fluid that is important for thinning semen after ejaculation to increase its likelihood of reaching the egg. The bulbourethral, or Cowper's, gland secretes an alkaline fluid that lubricates the urethra prior to ejaculation to neutralize any acidic urine residue.

The sperm along with all the exocrine secretions are collectively called semen. Their destination is the vagina and they can only get there if the penis is erect due to arousal and increased circulation. During sexual intercourse, ejaculation will forcefully expel the contents of the semen and effectively deliver the sperm to the egg. The muscular prostate gland is important for ejaculation. Each ejaculation releases 2 to 6 million sperm. Sperm has a whip-like flagellum tail that facilitates movement.

Female Reproductive System
The vagina is the passageway that sperm must travel through to reach an egg, the female gamete. Surrounding the vagina are the labia minor and labia major, both of which are folds that protect the urethra and the vaginal opening. The clitoris is rich in nerve-endings, making it sensitive and highly stimulated during sexual intercourse. It is above the vagina and urethra. An exocrine gland called the Bartholin's glands secretes a fluid during arousal that is important for lubrication.

The female gonads are the ovaries. Ovaries generally produce one immature gamete, an egg or oocyte, per month. They are also responsible for secreting the hormones estrogen and progesterone. Fertilization cannot happen unless the ejaculated sperm finds the egg, which are only available at certain times of the month. Eggs, or ova, develop in the ovaries in clusters surrounded by follicles, and after puberty, they are delivered to the uterus once a month via the fallopian tubes. The 28-day average journey of the egg to the uterus is called the menstrual cycle and it is highly regulated by the endocrine system. The regulatory hormones Gonadotropin releasing hormone (GnRH), luteinizing hormone (LH), and follicle-stimulating hormone (FSH) orchestrate the menstrual cycle. Ovarian hormones estrogen and progesterone are also important in timing as well as for vascularization of the uterus in preparation for pregnancy. Fertilization usually happens around ovulation, which is when the egg is inside the Fallopian tube. The resulting zygote travels down the tube and implants into the uterine wall. The uterus protects and nourishes the developing embryo for nine months until it is ready for the outside environment.

If the egg released is unfertilized, the uterine lining will slough off during menstruation. Should a fertilized egg, called a zygote, reach the uterus, it will embed itself into the uterine wall due to uterine vascularization that will deliver blood, nutrients, and antibodies to the developing embryo. The uterus is where the embryo will develop for the next nine months. Mammary glands are important female reproductive structures because they produce milk they provide for their young during lactation. Milk contains nutrients and antibodies that benefit the baby.

Anatomy and Physiology of the Integumentary System

The integumentary system includes skin, hair, nails, oil glands, and sweat glands. The largest organ of the integumentary system (and of the body), the skin, acts as a barrier and protects the body from mechanical impact, variations in temperature, microorganisms, chemicals, and UV radiation from the sun. It regulates body temperature, peripheral circulation, and excretes waste through sweat. It also contains a large network of nerve cells that relay changes in the external environment to the brain.

Layers of Skin

Skin consists of two layers, the surface epidermis and the inner dermis. The subcutaneous hypodermis is below the dermis and contains a layer of fat and connective tissue that are both important for insulation.

The whole epidermis is composed of epithelial cells that lack blood vessels. The outer epidermis is composed of dead cells which surround the living cells underneath. The most inner epidermal tissue is a single layer of cells called the stratum basale which is composed of rapidly dividing cells that push old cells to the skin's surface. When being pushed out, the cells' organelles disappear and they start producing a protein called keratin that eventually forms a tough waterproof layer. This outer layer sloughs off every four to five weeks. The melanocytes in the stratum basale produce the pigment melanin that absorbs UV rays and protects the skin. Skin also produces vitamin D if exposed to sunlight.

The dermis underneath the epidermis contains supporting collagen fibers peppered with nerves, blood vessels, hair follicles, sweat glands, oil glands, and smooth muscles.

Skin's Involvement in Temperature Homeostasis

The skin has a thermoregulatory role in the human body that is controlled by a negative feedback loop. The control center of temperature regulation is the hypothalamus in the brain. When the hypothalamus is alerted by receptors from the dermis, it secretes hormones that activate effectors to keep internal temperature at a set point of 98.6°F (37°C). If the environment is too cold, the hypothalamus will initiate a pathway that induces muscle shivering to release heat energy as well as constrict blood vessels to limit heat loss. In hot conditions, the hypothalamus will initiate a pathway that vasodilates blood vessels to increase heat loss and stimulate sweating for evaporative cooling. Evaporative cooling occurs when the hottest water particles evaporate and leave behind the coolest ones. This cools down the body.

Sebaceous Glands vs. Sweat Glands

The skin also contains oil glands, or sebaceous glands, and sweat glands that are exocrine because their substances are secreted through ducts. Endocrine glands secrete substances into the blood stream instead. Oil glands are attached to hair follicles. They secrete sebum, an oily substance that moisturizes the skin, protecting it from water loss. Sebum also keeps the skin elastic. Also, sebum's slight acidity provides a chemical defense against bacterial and fungal infections.

Sweat glands not attached to hair follicles are called eccrine glands. They are all over the body and these are the ones responsible for thermoregulation. They also remove bodily waste by secreting water and electrolytes. Sweat glands attached to hair follicles are apocrine glands and there are not nearly as many. Apocrine glands are only active post-puberty. They secrete a thicker, viscous substance that is attractive to bacteria, leading to the unpleasant smell in armpits, feet, and the groin. They are stimulated during stress and arousal.

Anatomy and Physiology of the Endocrine System

The endocrine system is made up of the ductless tissues and glands that secrete hormones directly into the bloodstream. It is similar to the nervous system in that it controls various functions of the body, but it does so via secretion of hormones in the bloodstream as opposed to nerve impulses. The endocrine system is also different because its effects last longer than that of the nervous system. Nerve impulses are immediate while hormone responses can last for minutes or even days.

The endocrine system works closely with the nervous system to regulate the physiological activities of the other systems of the body in order to maintain homeostasis. Hormone secretions are controlled by tight feedback loops that are generally regulated by the hypothalamus, the bridge between the nervous and endocrine systems. The hypothalamus receives sensory input via the nervous system and responds by stimulating or inhibiting the pituitary gland which stimulates or inhibits several other glands. The tight control is due to hormone secretions.

Hormones are chemicals that bind to specific target cells. Each hormone will only bind to a target cell that has a specific receptor that has the correct shape. For example, testosterone will not attach to skin cells because skin cells have no receptor that recognizes testosterone.

There are two types of hormones: steroid and protein. Steroid hormones are lipid, nonpolar substances, and most are able to diffuse across cell membranes. Once they do, they bind to a receptor that initiates a signal transduction cascade that affects gene expression. Non-steroid hormones bind to receptors on cell membranes that also initiate a signal transduction cascade that affects enzyme activity and chemical reactions.

Major Endocrine Glands

Hypothalamus: This gland is a part of the brain. It connects the nervous system to the endocrine system because it receives sensory information through nerves and it sends instructions via hormones delivered to the pituitary.

Pituitary Gland: This gland is pea-sized and is found at the bottom of the hypothalamus. It has two lobes called the anterior and posterior lobes. It plays an important role in regulating other endocrine glands. For example, it secretes growth hormone which regulates growth. Other hormones that are released by this gland control the reproductive system, childbirth, nursing, blood osmolarity, and metabolism.

The hormones and glands respond to each other via feedback loops, and a typical feedback loop is illustrated in the picture below. The hypothalamus and pituitary gland are master controllers of most of the other glands.

Thymus Gland: This gland is located in the chest cavity, embedded in connective tissue. It produces several hormones that are important for development and maintenance of T lymphocytes, which are important cells for immunity.

Adrenal Gland: One adrenal gland is attached to the top of each kidney. It produces epinephrine and norepinephrine which cause the "fight or flight" response in the face of danger or stress. These hormones raise heart rate, blood pressure, dilate bronchioles, and deliver blood to the muscles. All of these actions increase circulation and release glucose so that the body has an energy burst.

Pineal Gland: The pineal gland secretes melatonin, which is a hormone that regulates the body's circadian rhythms which are the natural wake-sleep cycles.

Testes and Ovaries: They secrete testosterone and both estrogen and progesterone, respectively. They are responsible for secondary sex characteristics, gamete development, and female hormones are important for embryonic development.

Thyroid Gland: This gland releases hormones like thyroxine and calcitonin. Thyroxine stimulates metabolism, and calcitonin monitors the amount of circulating calcium. Calcitonin signals the body to regulating calcium from bone reserves as well as kidney reabsorption of calcium.

Parathyroid Glands: These are four pea-sized glands located on the posterior surface of the thyroid. The main hormone that is secreted is called parathyroid hormone (PTH) which influences calcium levels like calcitonin, except it is antagonistic. PTH increases extracellular levels of calcium while calcitonin decreases it.

Pancreas: The pancreas is an organ that has both endocrine and exocrine functions. It functions outside of a typical feedback loop in that blood sugar seems to signal the pancreas itself n. The endocrine functions are controlled by the pancreatic islets of Langerhans, which are groups of beta cells scattered throughout the gland that secrete insulin to lower blood sugar levels in the body. Neighboring alpha cells secrete glucagon to raise blood sugar. These complementary hormones keep blood sugar in check.

Anatomy and Physiology of the Genitourinary System

The urinary system is made up of the kidneys, ureters, urinary bladder, and the urethra. It is the system responsible for removing waste products and balancing water and electrolyte concentrations in the blood. The urinary system has many important functions related to waste excretion. It regulates the concentrations of sodium, potassium, chloride, calcium, and other ions in the filtrate by controlling the amount of each that is reabsorbed during filtration. The reabsorption or secretion of hydrogen ions and bicarbonate contributes to the maintenance of blood pH. Certain kidney cells can detect any reductions in blood volume and pressure. If that happens, they secrete renin which will activate a hormone that causes increased reabsorption of sodium ions and water, raising volume and pressure. Under hypoxic conditions, kidney cells will secrete erythropoietin in order to stimulate red blood cell production. It also synthesizes calcitriol, which is a hormone derivative of vitamin D3 that aids in calcium ion absorption by the intestinal epithelium.

Under normal circumstances, humans have two functioning kidneys in the lower back and on either side of the spinal cord. They are the main organs that are responsible for filtering waste products out of the blood and regulating blood water and electrolyte levels. Blood enters the kidney through the renal artery and urea and wastes are removed while water and the acidity/alkalinity of the blood is adjusted. Toxic substances and drugs are also filtered. Blood exits through the renal vein and the urine waste travels through the ureter to the bladder where it is stored until it is eliminated through the urethra.

The kidneys have an outer renal cortex and an inner renal medulla that contain millions of tiny filtering units called nephrons. Nephrons have two parts: a glomerulus, which is the filter, and a tubule. The glomerulus is a network of capillaries covered by the Bowman's capsule, which is the entrance to the tubule. As blood enters the kidneys via the renal artery, the glomerulus allows for fluid and waste products to pass through it and enter the tubule. Blood cells and large molecules, such as proteins, do not pass through and remain in the blood. The filtrate passes through the tubule, which has several parts. The proximal tubule comes first, and then the descending and ascending limbs of the loop of Henle dip into the medulla, followed by the distal tubule and collecting duct. The journey through the tubule involves a balancing act that regulates blood osmolarity, pH, and electrolytes exchange of materials between the tubule and the blood stream. The final product at the collecting tubule is called urine, and it is delivered to the bladder by the ureter. The most central part of the kidney is the renal pelvis, and it acts as a funnel by delivering the urine from the millions of the collecting tubules to the ureters. The filtered blood exits through the renal vein and is returned to circulation.

Here's a look at the genitourinary system:

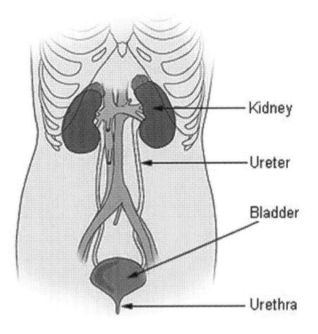

Here's a close up look at the kidney:

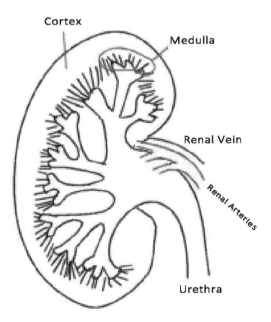

Waste Excretion
Once urine accumulates, it leaves the kidneys. The urine travels through the ureters into the urinary bladder, a muscular organ that is hollow and elastic. As more urine enters the urinary bladder, its walls stretch and become thinner so there is no significant difference in internal pressure. The urinary bladder stores the urine until the

body is ready for urination, at which time the muscles contract and force the urine through the urethra and out of the body.

Anatomy and Physiology of the Immune System

The immune system is the body's offense against invading microorganisms (bacteria, viruses, fungi, and parasites) and other harmful, foreign substances. It is capable of limiting or preventing infection.

There are two general types of immunity: innate immunity and acquired immunity. Innate immunity uses physical and chemical barriers to block microorganism entry into the body. The biggest barrier is the skin; it forms a physical barrier that blocks microorganisms from entering underlying tissues. Mucous membranes in the digestive, respiratory, and urinary systems secrete mucus to block and remove invading microorganisms. Other natural defenses include saliva, tears, and stomach acids, which are all chemical barriers intended to block infection with microorganisms. Acid is inhospitable to pathogens, as are tears, mucus, and saliva which all contain a natural antibiotic called lysozyme. The respiratory passages contain microscopic cilia which are like bristles that sweep out pathogens. In addition, macrophages and other white blood cells can recognize and eliminate foreign objects through phagocytosis or toxic secretions.

Acquired immunity refers to a specific set of events used by the body to fight a particular infection. Essentially, the body accumulates and stores information about the nature of an invading microorganism. As a result, the body can mount a specific attack that is much more effective than innate immunity. It also provides a way for the body to prevent future infections by the same microorganism.

Acquired immunity is divided into a primary response and a secondary response. The primary immune response occurs the first time a particular microorganism enters the body, where macrophages engulf the microorganism and travel to the lymph nodes. In the lymph nodes, macrophages present the invader to helper T lymphocytes, which then activate humoral and cellular immunity. Humoral immunity refers to immunity resulting from antibody production by B lymphocytes. After being activated by helper T lymphocytes, B lymphocytes multiply and divide into plasma cells and memory cells. Plasma cells are B lymphocytes that produce immune proteins called antibodies, or immunoglobulins. Antibodies then bind the microorganism to flag it for destruction by other white blood cells. Cellular immunity refers to the immune response coordinated by T lymphocytes. After being activated by helper T lymphocytes, other T lymphocytes attack and kill cells that cause infection or disease.

The secondary immune response takes place during subsequent encounters with a known microorganism. Memory cells respond to the previously encountered microorganism by immediately producing antibodies. Memory cells are B lymphocytes that store information to produce antibodies. The secondary immune response is swift and powerful, because it eliminates the need for the time-consuming macrophage activation of the primary immune response. Suppressor T lymphocytes also take part to inhibit the immune response as an overactive immune response could cause damage to healthy cells.

Inflammation occurs if a pathogen evades the barriers and chemical defenses. It stimulates pain receptors, alerting the individual that something is wrong. It also elevates body temperature to speed up chemical reactions, although if a fever goes unchecked it can be dangerous due to the fact that extreme heat unfolds proteins. Histamine is secreted which dilates blood vessels and recruits white blood cells that destroy invaders non-specifically. The immune system is tied to the lymphatic system. The thymus, one of the lymphatic system organs, is the site of maturation of T-cells, a type of white blood cell. The lymphatic system is important in the inflammatory response because lymph vessels deliver leukocytes and collect debris that will be filtered in the lymph nodes and the spleen.

Antigen and Typical Immune Response

Should a pathogen evade barriers and survive through inflammation, an antigen-specific adaptive immune response will begin. Immune cells recognize these foreign particles by their antigens, which are their unique and identifying surface proteins. Drugs, toxins, and transplanted cells can also act as antigens. The body even recognizes its own cells as potential threats in autoimmune diseases.

When a macrophage engulfs a pathogen and presents its antigens, helper T cells recognize the signal and secrete cytokines to signal T lymphocytes and B lymphocytes so that they launch the cell-mediated and humoral response, respectively. The cell-mediated response occurs when the T lymphocytes kill infected cells by secreting cytotoxins. The humoral response occurs when B lymphocytes proliferate into plasma and memory cells. The plasma cells secrete antigen-specific antibodies which bind to the pathogens so that they cannot bind to host cells. Macrophages and other phagocytic cells called neutrophils engulf and degrade the antibody/pathogen complex. The memory cells remain in circulation and initiate a secondary immune response should the pathogen dare enter the host again.

Active and Passive Immunity

Acquired immunity occurs after the first antigen encounter. The first time the body mounts this immune response is called the primary immune response. Because the memory B cells store information about the antigen's structure, any subsequent immune response causes a secondary immune response which is much faster and substantially more antibodies are produced due to the presence of memory B cells. If the secondary immune response is strong and fast enough, it will fight off the pathogen before an individual becomes symptomatic. This is a natural means of acquiring immunity.

Vaccination is the process of inducing immunity. *Active immunization* refers to immunity gained by exposure to infectious microorganisms or viruses and can be *natural* or *artificial*. Natural immunization refers to an individual being exposed to an infectious organism as a part of daily life. For example, it was once common for parents to expose their children to childhood diseases such as measles or chicken pox. Artificial immunization refers to therapeutic exposure to an infectious organism as a way of protecting an individual from disease. Today, the medical community relies on artificial immunization as a way to induce immunity.

Vaccines are used for the development of active immunity. A vaccine contains a killed, weakened, or inactivated microorganism or virus that is administered through injection, by mouth, or by aerosol. Vaccinations are administered to prevent an infectious disease but do not always guarantee immunity. Due to circulating memory B cells after administration, the secondary response will fight off the pathogen should it be encountered again in many cases. Both illness and vaccinations cause active immunity.

Passive immunity refers to immunity gained by the introduction of antibodies. This introduction can be also be natural or artificial. The process occurs when antibodies from the mother's bloodstream are passed on to the bloodstream of the developing fetus. Breast milk can also transmit antibodies to a baby. Babies are born with passive immunity, which provides protection against general infection for approximately the first six months of its life.

<u>Types of Leukocytes</u>
There are many leukocytes, or white blood cells, involved in both innate and adaptive immunity. All are developed in bone marrow. Many have been mentioned in the text above, but a comprehensive list is included here for reference.

- Monocytes are large phagocytic cells.
  - Macrophages engulf pathogens and present their antigen. Some circulate, but others reside in lymphatic organs like the spleen and lymph nodes.
  - Dendritic cells are also phagocytic and antigen-presenting.

- Granulocytes are cells that contain secretory granules.
  - Neutrophils are the most abundant white blood cell. They are circulating and aggressive phagocytic cells that are part of innate immunity. They also secrete substances that are toxic to pathogens.
  - Basophils and mast cells secrete histamine which stimulates the inflammatory response.
  - Eosinophils are found underneath mucous membranes and defend against multi-cellular parasites like worms. They have low phagocytic activity and primarily secrete destructive enzymes.
- T lymphocytes mature in the thymus.
  - Helper T cells recognize antigens presented by macrophages and dendritic cells and secrete cytokines that mount the humoral and cell-mediated immune response.
  - Killer T cells are cytotoxic cells involved in the cell-mediated response by recognizing and poisoning infected cells.
  - Suppressor T cells suppress the adaptive immune response when there is no threat to conserve resources and energy.
  - Memory T cells remain in circulation to aid in the secondary immune response.
- B lymphocytes mature in bone marrow.
  - Plasma B cells secrete antigen-specific antibodies when signaled by Helper T cells and are degraded after the immune response.
  - Memory B cells store antigen-specific antibody making instructions and remain circulating after the immune response is over.
- Natural killer cells are part of innate immunity and patrol and identify suspect-material. They respond by secreting cytotoxic substances.

Anatomy and Physiology of the Skeletal System

<u>Axial Skeleton and Appendicular Skeleton</u>
The skeletal system is composed of 206 bones interconnected by tough connective tissue called ligaments. The axial skeleton can be considered the north-south axis of the skeleton. It includes the spinal column, sternum, ribs, and skull. There are 80 bones in the axial skeleton, and 33 of them are vertebrae. The ribs make up 12 of the bones in the axial skeleton.

The remaining 126 bones are in the appendicular skeleton which contains bones of the appendages like the collarbone (clavicle), shoulders (scapula), arms, hands, hips, legs, and feet. The arm bones consist of the upper humerus with the radius and ulna that attach to the hands. The wrists, hands, and fingers are composed of the carpals, metacarpals, and phalanges, respectively. The femur attaches to the hips. The patella or kneecap connects the femur to the fibula and tibia. The ankles, feet, and toes are composed of the tarsals, metatarsals, and phalanges, respectively.

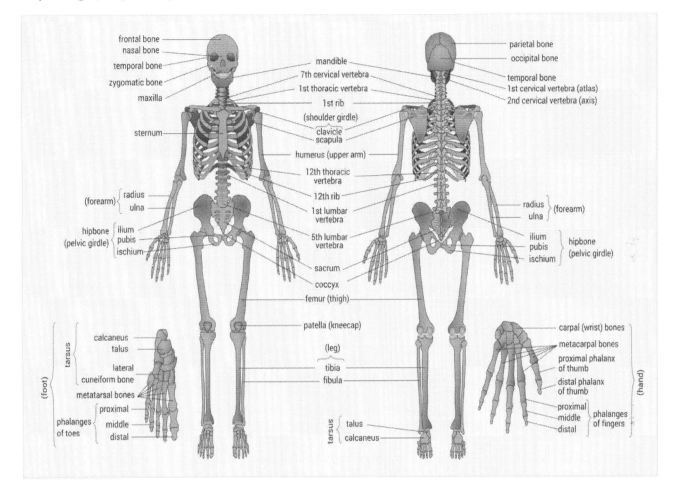

Functions of the Skeletal System

One of the skeletal system's most important functions is to protect vital internal organs. The skull protects the brain, the ribs protect the lungs and heart, the vertebrae protect the spinal column, and the pelvis protects the uterus and other reproductive organs. Yellow bone marrow stores lipids, or fats, and red bone marrow produces red and white blood cells as well as platelets. The bones themselves store the essential minerals calcium and phosphorous. The organization of the skeleton allows us to stand upright and acts as a foundation for organs and tissues to attach and maintain their location. This is similar to how the wooden frame of a house has room partitions to designate the type of room and floors that furniture can attach to.

The skeletal system and the muscular system are literally interconnected and allow for voluntary movement. Strong connective tissues called tendons attach bones to muscles. Most muscles work in opposing pairs and act as levers. For example, flexing the biceps brings the arm bones together and flexing the triceps pushes them apart. Synovial joints are movable joints, and they are rich with cartilage, connective tissue, and synovial fluid which acts as a lubricant. The majority of joints are synovial joints, and they include hinge joints, like the one at the elbow, which allows for opening and closing.

The vertebrae are cartilaginous joints which have spaces between them filled with cushion-like discs that act as shock absorbers and glue that holds the vertebrae together. The reason for the tight packing of the vertebrae is to protect the spinal cord inside. This limits their movement, but because there are so many of them it allows the backbone to be flexible.

Fibrous joints like those in the skull have fibrous tissue between the bones and no cavity between them. These are fixed joints that are immobile.

Compact and Spongy Bone

Osteoclasts, osteoblasts, and osteocytes are the three types of bone cells. Osteoclasts break down old bone, osteoblasts make new bone, and osteocytes are the mature functional bone cells. Bone is constantly regenerating due to the osteoblasts/osteoclasts that line all types of bones and the blood vessels inside them. The cells all exist within a matrix of collagen fibers that provide resistance to tension and minerals that provide resistance to compression. Because of the collagen and mineral matrix, bones have ample reinforcement to collectively support the entire human body.

Bones can be classified as any of the following:

- Long bones include tube-like rods like the arm and leg bones.
- Short bones are tube-like rods that are smaller than long bones like the fingers and toes.
- Flat bones are thin and flat like the ribs and breastbone.
- Irregular bones like the vertebrae are compact and don't fit into the other categories.

The outer tissue of the bone is surrounded by connective tissue known as periosteum. It appears shiny, smooth, and white. It protects the bone, anchors the bone to the connective tissue that surrounds muscles, and links the bone to the circulatory and nervous system. Compact bone is underneath the periosteum and is made of a dense blend of tightly packed osteocytes a mineral reservoir of calcium and phosphorous. Compact bones have a Haversian system that is composed of embedded blood vessels, lymph vessels, and nerve bundles that span the interior of the bone from one end to the other. Branching from the central canal to the surface of the bone are the canals of Volkmann which deliver materials to peripheral osteocytes. Concentric circles surround the central Haversian canal, and these lamallae have gaps between them called lacunae where osteocytes are embedded.

In contrast, spongy bone is very porous and more flexible than compact bone. It is at the ends of long bones and the central part of flat bones. It looks like a honeycomb, and the open spaces are connected by trabeculae which are beams of tissue that add support. They add strength without adding mass.

Cartilage is a very flexible connective tissue made of collagen and the flexible elastin. It has no blood vessels and obtains materials via diffusion. It is replaced by bone starting in infancy in a process called ossification.

Life and Physical Sciences

Basic Macromolecules in a Biological System

There are four classes of macromolecules that allow organisms to exist: carbohydrates, lipids, proteins, and nucleic acids. Carbon is the backbone of these organic molecules because of its ability to form up to four covalent bonds. Carbon (C), hydrogen (H), oxygen (O), nitrogen (N), sulfur (S), and phosphorus (P) are the most prevalent elements in these biological molecules. The following chart gives an overview of each organic molecule.

Organic Molecule	Example	Monomer (smallest repeating unit)	Structure	Function
Carbohydrate	• Sugar • Cellulose	Monosaccharide	Glucose Fructose Galactose	• Energy • Structure
Protein	• Actin • Insulin	Amino Acid		• Structure • Support • Some hormones
Lipid	• Fat • Oil	Technically none because the glycerol and fatty acids are not repeating.	Glycerol Triglyceride-Saturated	• Long-term energy • Steroid Hormones • Cell membranes

Organic Molecule	Example	Monomer (smallest repeating unit)	Structure	Function
Nucleic Acid	• DNA • RNA	Nucleotide	Phosphate group / NITROGENOUS BASE (e.g. Adenine) / SUGAR (Deoxyribose or Ribose)	• Genetic code • Makes Protein

Carbohydrates

Carbohydrates are usually sweet, ring-like sugar molecules that are built from carbon (carbo-) and oxygen & hydrogen (-hydrates, meaning water). They can exist as one-ring monosaccharides, like glucose, fructose, and galactose, or as two-ring disaccharides, like lactose, maltose, and sucrose. These simple sugars can be easily broken down and used via glycolysis to provide a source of quick energy. Polysaccharides are repeating chains of monosaccharide rings. They are more complex carbohydrates, and there are several types. For example:

- Plants store energy in the form of *starch*.
- Animals store energy in the form of *glycogen*. Vertebrates store glycogen in the liver and in muscle cells.
- *Cellulose* is the chief structural component of plant cell walls.
- *Chitin* is the chief structural component of fungi cell walls and the exoskeletons of arthropods.

Proteins

Proteins are composed of chains of amino acids. There are several different kinds.

- Enzymes catalyze chemical reactions in the body.
- Storage proteins like albumin in eggs are important for development.
- Hormonal proteins are responsible for initiating signal transduction cascades that regulate gene expression.
- Motor proteins like actin and myosin are responsible for movement.
- Immune proteins like antibodies and antigens are important for fighting disease.
- Transport proteins like channel proteins and protein pumps move molecules.
- Receptor proteins receive chemical messages like neurotransmitters.
- Marker proteins serve as a cell's identification or fingerprint that distinguishes between cells of different types and sources.
- Structural proteins like keratin are important for things like spider webs, hair, and feathers.

All proteins are made from a combination of 20 amino acids. The varying amino acids are linked by peptide bonds and form the primary structure of the polypeptide, or chain of amino acids. The primary structure is just the string of amino acids. It is the secondary, tertiary, and quaternary structure that determines protein shape and function. The secondary structure can be beta sheets or alpha helices formed by hydrogen bonding between the polar regions of the polypeptide backbone. Tertiary structure results from the interactions between the side chains. Quaternary structure is the overall protein structure that occurs when subunits merge, take the correct shape, and become functional.

Lipids

Lipids are mostly nonpolar, hydrophobic molecules that are not soluble in water. Triglycerides are a type of lipid with a glycerol backbone attached to three long fatty acid chains. These energy-storage molecules can exist as any of the following types.

- Saturated fats have no double bonds within their fatty acid tails. These are solid at room temperature and are mostly animal fats like bacon fat.

- Unsaturated fats have double bonds within any of their fatty acid tails. Due to the kinks caused by the double bonds, these fats are liquid at room temperature and are mostly plant fats like olive oil.

Phospholipids are also composed of glycerol except they have two fatty acid tails. The third tail is replaced with a hydrophilic phosphate group. The amphipathic nature of this molecule results in a lipid bilayer where the "water-loving" hydrophilic heads face the extracellular matrix and cytoplasm and the "water-hating" hydrophobic tails face each other on the inside.

Steroids are another type of lipid. Cholesterol is a steroid that embeds itself in animal cell membranes and acts as a fluidity buffer. Steroid hormones such as testosterone and estrogen are responsible for transcriptional regulation in certain cells.

Nucleic acids

Nucleic acids are made of nucleotides. Nucleotides consist of a five-carbon sugar, a nitrogen-containing base, and a phosphate group. Deoxyribonucleic acid (DNA) exists as two nucleotide chains arranged in a double helix. Each deoxyribose sugar is connected to a nitrogen base and an electrically negative phosphate group. The nitrogen bases are adenine and guanine, the two-ringed purines, and cytosine and thymine, the one-ringed pyrimidines. The double helix is held together by weak hydrogen bonds that connect adenine to thymine and cytosine to guanine. Ribonucleic acid (RNA) has a slightly different structure. It is usually single-stranded, has a ribose sugar as opposed to deoxyribose, and contains uracil instead of thymine.

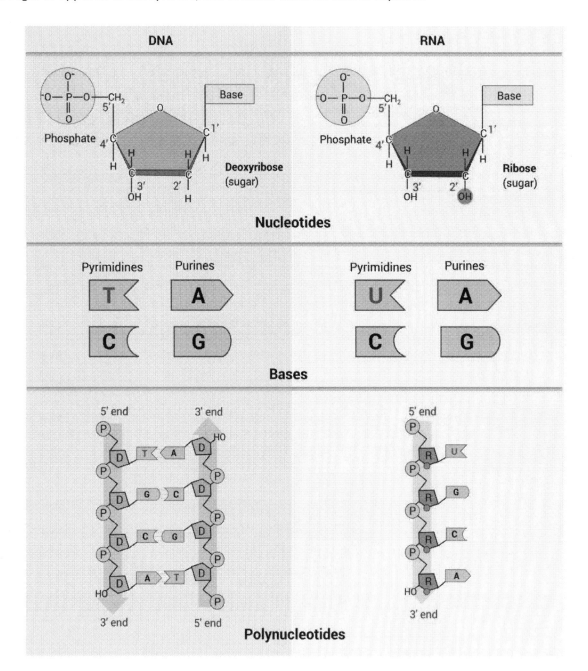

160

DNA forms the genetic code in the nucleus of eukaryotes, and RNA is the interpreter that comes in many varieties.

- Messenger RNA (mRNA) copies the DNA into a complementary transcript. This process is called *transcription*.
- Ribosomal RNA (rRNA) makes up the protein-making structure called the ribosome which reads the transcript in a process called *translation*.
- Transfer RNA (tRNA) carries amino acids and delivers them to the ribosome. Each three letters of the mRNA transcript, or codon, recruits the anti-codon of a tRNA molecule that carries the corresponding amino acid.

Comparing and Contrasting Chromosomes, Genes, and DNA

Nucleic Acids
Nucleic acids have two important duties in the body. As monomers, they are crucial for energy transfer. As polymers, they are a fundamental component of genetic material. Monomers are the simplest form of a biochemical, while polymers are the complex form of a biochemical.

Nucleotides are used to assemble nucleic acids. Nucleotides have three components: a nitrogen base and a phosphate functional group both attached to a five-carbon (pentose) sugar. There are two classes of nitrogen bases, purines and pyrimidines. The two types of purines are guanine (G) and adenine (A) while the three types of pyrimidines are thymine (T), cytosine (C), and uracil (U). The two types of pentose sugars are deoxyribose and ribose. Nucleotides containing deoxyribose are termed deoxyribonucleic acids (DNA) and utilize guanine, adenine, cytosine, and thymine as its nitrogen bases. Nucleotides containing ribose are termed ribonucleic acids (RNA) and utilize guanine, adenine, cytosine, and uracil as its nitrogen bases.

Chromosomes are composed of hundreds to thousands of genes. Human cells contain 23 pairs of chromosomes for a total of 46 chromosomes. As explained above, genes are inherited in pairs, one from each parent.

Proteins are made of long chains of amino acids. In total, there are 20 amino acids, 11 of which humans can synthesize on their own and the remaining 9 of which are procured through diet. DNA contains the information for the synthesis of proteins, but that information on DNA has to undergo transcription and translation by RNA in order to produce proteins.

Codons
A codon represents a sequence of three nucleotides, which codes for either one specific amino acid or a stop signal during protein synthesis. Codons are found on messenger RNA (mRNA).

20 essential amino acids are utilized in the process of protein synthesis. The full set of codons encompasses 64 possible combinations and is termed the genetic code. In the genetic code, 61 codons represent amino acids and three codons are stop signals. The genetic code is redundant due to the fact that a single amino acid may be produced by multiple codons. For example, the codons AAA and AAG produce the amino acid lysine. The codons UAA, UAG, and UGA are stop signals. The codon AUG codes for both the amino acid methionine and the start signal. As a result, AUG when found in mRNA marks the initiation point of protein translation.

RNA
Ribonucleic acid (RNA) plays crucial roles in protein synthesis and gene regulation. RNA is made of nucleotides consisting of ribose (a sugar), a phosphate group, and one of four possible nitrogen bases—adenine (A), cytosine (C), guanine (G), and uracil (U). RNA utilizes the nitrogen base uracil in place of the base thymine found in DNA. Another difference between RNA and DNA is that RNA is typically found as a single-stranded structure, while DNA typically exists in a double-stranded structure.

RNA can be categorized into three major groups—messenger RNA (mRNA), ribosomal RNA (rRNA), and transfer RNA (tRNA). Messenger RNA (mRNA) transports instructions from DNA in the nucleus of a cell to the areas responsible for protein synthesis in the cytoplasm of a cell. This process is known as transcription. Transfer RNA (tRNA) deciphers the amino acid sequence for the construction of proteins found in mRNA. Both tRNA and ribosomal RNA (rRNA) are found in the ribosomes of cells. Ribosomes are responsible for protein synthesis. The process is also known as translation and both tRNA and rRNA play crucial roles. Both translation and transcription are further described below.

DNA

Deoxyribonucleic acid, or DNA, contains the genetic material that is passed from parent to offspring. It contains specific instructions for the development and function of a unique eukaryotic organism. The great majority of cells in a eukaryotic organism contains the same DNA.

The majority of DNA can be found in the cell's nucleus and is referred to as nuclear DNA. A small amount of DNA can be located in the mitochondria and is referred to as mitochondrial DNA. Mitochondria provide the energy for a properly functioning cell. All offspring inherit mitochondrial DNA from their mother. James Watson, an American geneticist, and Frances Crick, a British molecular biologist, first outlined the structure of DNA in 1953.

The structure of DNA visually approximates a twisting ladder and is described as a double helix. DNA is made of nucleotides consisting of deoxyribose (a sugar), a phosphate group, and one of four possible nitrogen bases— thymine (T), adenine (A), cytosine (C), and guanine (G). It is estimated that human DNA contains three billion bases. The sequence of these bases dictates the instructions contained in the DNA making each species singular. The bases in DNA pair in a particular manner—thymine (T) with adenine (A) and guanine (G) with cytosine (C). Weak hydrogen bonds amongst the nitrogen bases ensure easy uncoiling of DNA's double helical structure in preparation for replication.

Transcription

Transcription refers to a portion of DNA being copied into RNA, specifically mRNA. It represents the first crucial step in gene expression. The process begins with the enzyme RNA polymerase binding to the promoter region of DNA, which initiates transcription of a specific gene. RNA polymerase then untwists the double helix of DNA by breaking weak hydrogen bonds between its nucleotides. Once DNA is untwisted, RNA polymerase travels down the strand reading the DNA sequence and adding complementary nitrogen bases. With the assistance of RNA polymerase, the pentose sugar and phosphate functional group are added to the nitrogen base to form a nucleotide. Lastly, the weak hydrogen bonds uniting the DNA-RNA complex are broken to free the newly formed mRNA. The mRNA travels from the nucleus of the cell out to the cytoplasm of the cell where translation occurs.

Translation

Translation refers to the process of ribosomes synthesizing proteins. It represents the second crucial step in gene expression. The instructions encoding specific proteins to be made are contained in codons on mRNA, which have previously been transcribed from DNA. Each codon represents a specific amino acid or stop signal in the genetic code.

Amino acids are the building blocks of proteins. Ribosomes contain transfer RNA (tRNA) and ribosomal RNA (rRNA). Translation occurs in ribosomes located in the cytoplasm of cells and consists of the following three phases:

Initiation: The ribosome gathers at a target point on the mRNA, and tRNA attaches at the start codon (AUG), which is also the codon for the amino acid methionine.

Elongation: A new tRNA reads the next codon on the mRNA and links the two amino acids together with a peptide bond. The process is repeated until a polypeptide, or long chain of amino acids, is formed.

Termination: The ribosome disengages from the mRNA when it encounters a stop codon (UAA, UAG, or UGA). The event releases the polypeptide molecule. Proteins are made of one or more polypeptide molecules.

Explaining Mendel's Laws of Heredity

Genes are the basis of heredity. The German scientist Gregor Mendel first suggested the existence of genes in 1866. A gene can be pinpointed to a locus, or a particular position, on DNA. It is estimated that humans have approximately 20,000 to 25,000 genes. For any particular gene, a human inherits one copy from each parent for a total of two.

Genotype refers to the genetic makeup of an individual within a species. Phenotype refers to the visible characteristics and observable behavior of an individual within a species.

Genotypes are written with pairs of letters that represent alleles. Alleles are different versions of the same gene, and, in simple systems, each gene has one dominant allele and one recessive allele. The letter of the dominant trait is capitalized, while the letter of the recessive trait is not capitalized. An individual can be homozygous dominant, homozygous recessive, or heterozygous for a particular gene. *Homozygous* means that the individual inherits two alleles of the same type while *heterozygous* means inheriting one dominant allele and one recessive allele.

If an individual has homozygous dominant alleles or heterozygous alleles, the dominant allele is expressed. If an individual has homozygous recessive alleles, the recessive allele is expressed. For example, a species of bird develops either white or black feathers. The white feathers are the dominant allele, or trait (*A*), while the black feathers are the recessive allele (*a*). Homozygous dominant (*AA*) and heterozygous (*Aa*) birds will develop white feathers. Homozygous recessive (aa) birds will develop black feathers.

Genotype (genetic makeup)	Phenotype (observable traits)
AA	white feathers
Aa	white feathers
aa	black feathers

<u>Influence of Phenotype on Genotype</u>
The genetic material (DNA) inherited from an individual's parents determines genotype. Natural selection leads to adaptations within a species, which affects the phenotype. Over time, individuals within a species with the most advantageous phenotypes will survive and reproduce. As result of reproduction, the subsequent generation of phenotypes receives the fittest genotype. Eventually, the individuals within a species with genetic fitness flourish and those without it are erased from the environment. As explained above, this is also referred to as the concept of "survival of the fittest". When this process is duplicated over numerous generations, the outcome is offspring with a level of genetic fitness that meets or exceeds that of their parents.

<u>Mendel's Laws of Genetics and Punnett Squares</u>
Mendel's first law of genetics is the principle of *segregation* and states that alleles will segregate into different cells during the formation of gametes in meiosis. Mendel's second law of genetics is the principle of *independent*

assortment and states that genes for different traits will be assigned to different gametes independent of the others. Together, these two laws state the assumptions on which genetic probabilities are based.

Punnett squares are simple graphic representations of all the possible genotypes of offspring, given the genotypes of the parent organisms. For instance, in the above example with the species of bird with black or white feathers, *A* represents a dominant allele and determines white colored feathers on a bird. The recessive allele *a* determines black colored feathers on a bird. If both parents are heterozygous (*Aa*, the x and y axis of the square) the offspring will have the possible genotypes *AA*, *Aa*, *Aa*, and *aa*. Phenotypically, three offspring would have white feathers and one would have black feathers, as shown in the below Punnett square.

Monohybrid and Dihybrid Genetic Crosses
Genetic crosses represent all possible permutations of gene combinations, or alleles. A monohybrid cross investigates the inheritance pattern of a single gene such as in the above example of the birds with black or white feathers. Both parents must have heterozygous gene pairs in a monohybrid cross.

The phenotypic ratio for a monohybrid cross is 3:1 (*AA*, *Aa*, *Aa*, *aa*) in favor of the dominant gene. A dihybrid cross investigates the inheritance patterns of two genes that are related, for example *A* and *B*. A dihybrid cross has a phenotypic ratio of 9:3:3:1 with nine offspring inheriting both dominant genes, six offspring inheriting a single dominant and a single recessive gene, and one offspring inheriting both recessive genes.

Recognizing Basic Atomic Structure

Measurable Properties of Atoms
All matter is made of atoms. Atoms are the most basic portion of an element that still retains its properties. All of the elements known to man are catalogued in the periodic table, a chart of elements arranged by increasing atomic number. The atomic number refers to the number of protons in an atom's nucleus. It can be found either in the upper left hand corner of the box or directly above an element's chemical symbol on the periodic table. For example, the atomic number for hydrogen (H) is 1. The term "atomic mass" refers to the sum of protons and neutrons in an atom's nucleus. The atomic mass can be found beneath an element's abbreviation on the periodic table. For example, the average atomic mass of hydrogen (H) is 1.008. Because protons have a positive charge and neutrons have a neutral charge, an atom's nucleus typically has a positive electrical charge. Electrons orbiting the nucleus have a negative charge. As a result, elements with equal numbers of protons and electrons have no net charge.

Atoms that have gained or lost electrons wind up having a net electrical charge and are termed ions. The following are the main ions related to human health:

Bicarbonate	HCO^{3-}	A major buffer in blood. The lungs and kidneys regulate its concentration.
Chloride	Cl^-	Important in stomach acid and usually ingested as the salts sodium chloride (NaCl) and potassium chloride (KCl).
Calcium	Ca^{2+}	Important to muscle contraction and bone construction.
Copper	Cu	Specialized chemical reactions in the cell.
Iodine	I	Specialized chemical reactions in the cell.
Iron	Fe	Important in hemoglobin for transport of oxygen as well as part of the electron transport chain.
Magnesium	Mg^{2+}	Important in chlorophyll and animal energy production as well as a constituent of bone.
Phosphate	PO_4^{3-}	A minor intracellular pH buffer that is regulated by the kidneys and is an important factor in bone.
Potassium	K^+	The most plentiful mineral inside of cells and is important for nerve and muscle function.
Sodium	Na^+	The most common mineral outside of cells and is important for water and osmolarity regulation as well as nerve and muscle function.
Sulfate	SO_4^{2-}	A minor pH buffer for body fluids.

For the majority of light atoms, the number of protons is similar to the number of neutrons. An isotope is a variation of an element having the same number of protons, but a different number of neutrons. For example, all isotopes of carbon (C) have six protons. Nevertheless, C-12 has six neutrons, C-13 has seven neutrons, and C-14 has eight neutrons.

Some isotopes are radioactive and result in nuclear decay. Not all radioactive isotopes are harmful, and some are even useful to scientists and physicians. For example, C-14 is radioactive and can be used in the process of radiocarbon dating, which can be used to determine the age of organic remains. A radioactive isotope of gold (Au-198) can be utilized to treat ovarian, prostate, and brain cancer.

Periodicity and the Periodic Table
Periodicity
Periodicity refers to the repeating patterns, or trends, in the properties of elements. The atomic number and atomic structure are the key determinants of the properties of elements. During the mid-1800s, the Russian chemist Dmitri Mendeleev utilized the principal of periodicity to arrange elements in a manner similar to the modern periodic table. Mendeleev's periodic table was arranged in rows according to increasing atomic mass and in columns according to similar chemical behavior. The modern periodic table is arranged in order of increasing atomic number, which is defined as the number of protons in an atom's nucleus. Elements near each other are more similar than elements that are distant on the periodic table.

Periodic Table
The periodic table catalogues all of the elements known to man, currently 118. It is one of the most important references in the science of chemistry. Information that can be gathered from the periodic table includes the element's atomic number, atomic mass, and chemical symbol. The first periodic table was rendered by Mendeleev in the mid-1800s and was ordered according to increasing atomic mass. The modern periodic table is arranged in order of increasing atomic number. It is also arranged in horizontal rows known as periods, and vertical columns known as families, or groups. The periodic table contains seven periods and eighteen families. Elements in the periodic table can also be classified into three major groups: metals, metalloids, and nonmetals. Metals are concentrated on the left side of the periodic table, while nonmetals are found on the right side. Metalloids occupy the area between the metals and nonmetals.

Due to the fact the periodic table is ordered by increasing atomic number, the electron configurations of the elements show periodicity. As the atomic number increases, electrons gradually fill the shells of an atom. In general, the start of a new period corresponds to the first time an electron inhabits a new shell. Other trends in the properties of elements in the periodic table are:

Atomic radius: One-half the distance between the nuclei of atoms of the same element.

Electronegativity: A measurement of the willingness of an atom to form a chemical bond.

Ionization energy: The amount of energy needed to remove an electron from a gas or ion.

Electron affinity: The ability of an atom to accept an electron.

Moving left to right in a period, trends reveal decreasing atomic radius, increasing electronegativity, increasing ionization energy, and increasing electron affinity. Moving from top to bottom in a group, trends reveal increasing atomic radius, decreasing electronegativity, and decreasing ionization energy. The trend of decreasing electron affinity is only seen in Group 1 of the periodic table.

Protons, Neutrons, and Electrons
The structure of an atom has two major components: the atomic nucleus and the atomic shells. The nucleus is found in the center of an atom. The three major subatomic particles are protons, neutrons, and electrons and are found in the atomic nucleus and shells.

Protons are found in the atomic nucleus and are positively charged particles. The addition or removal of protons from an atom's nucleus creates an entirely different element. *Neutrons* are also found in the atomic nucleus and are neutral particles, meaning they have no net electrical charge. The addition or removal of neutrons from an atom's nucleus does not create a different element but instead creates a lighter or heavier form of that element called an isotope. *Electrons* are found orbiting in the atomic shells around the nucleus and are negatively charged particles. A proton or a neutron has nearly 2,000 times the mass of an electron.

Electrons and Chemical Bonds
Electrons orbit the nucleus in atomic shells. For example, the first atomic shell can accommodate two electrons, the second atomic shell can hold a maximum of eight electrons, and the third atomic shell can house a maximum of eight electrons. The negatively charged electrons orbiting the nucleus are attracted to the positively charged protons in the nucleus via electromagnetic force. The attraction of opposite electrical charges gives rise to chemical bonds, which refers to the ways atoms are attached to each other.

Chemical bonding typically results in the formation of a new substance. Only the electrons in the outermost atomic shell are able to form chemical bonds. These electrons are known as valence electrons, and they are what determines the chemical properties of an atom.

Chemical Bonds Between Atoms

Chemical bonds refer to the manner in which atoms are attached to one another. Atoms may be held together with three fundamental types of chemical bonds—ionic, covalent, or hydrogen.

Ionic Bonding

Ionic bonds are formed from the electrostatic attractions between oppositely charged atoms. They result from the transfer of electrons from a metal on the left side of the periodic table to a nonmetal on the right side. In an *ionic bond*, an atom loses one or more electrons to another who gains them. The atoms do this so that they can achieve a full outermost shell of electrons, which is the configuration with the lowest amount of energy, and these are typically the strongest types of bonds. The metallic substance often has a low ionization energy and will transfer an electron easily to the nonmetal, which has a high electron affinity. An example of this is the compound NaCl, which is sodium chloride or table salt, where the Na atom transfers an electron to the Cl atom. Due to their very strong bonding, ionic compounds have several distinct characteristics. They have high melting points and high boiling points, and are brittle and crystalline. They are arranged in rigid, well-defined structures, which allows them to break apart along smooth, flat surfaces. The formation of ionic bonds is a reaction that is very exothermic. In the opposite scenario, the energy it takes to break up a one mole quantity of an ionic compound is referred to as lattice energy, which is generally very endothermic. The Lewis structure for NaCl is written as follows:

$$Na + \cdot\overset{\displaystyle\cdot\cdot}{\underset{\displaystyle\cdot\cdot}{Cl}}{:} \rightarrow Na^+ + {:}\overset{\displaystyle\cdot\cdot}{\underset{\displaystyle\cdot\cdot}{Cl}}{:}^-$$

When an atom has a different number of electrons than its number of protons, it is termed an *ion*. A positively charged ion is referred to as a *cation*, while a negatively charged ion is referred to as an *anion*. For example, a sodium cation (Na^{+1}) can form an ionic bond to a chlorine anion (Cl^{-1}) to form sodium chloride (NaCl), which is also known as table salt. The majority of the molecules formed with ionic bonds such as this have a crystalline structure.

Covalent Bonding

Covalent bonds are formed when two atoms share electrons, instead of transferring them like in ionic compounds. The atoms in covalent compounds have a balance of attraction and repulsion between their protons and electrons, which keeps them bonded together. Two atoms can be joined by single, double, or even triple covalent bonds. As the number of electrons that are shared increases, the length of the bond decreases. Covalent substances have low melting and boiling points and are also poor conductors of heat and electricity. The Lewis structure for Cl_2 is written as follows:

$$\cdot\overset{\displaystyle\cdot\cdot}{\underset{\displaystyle\cdot\cdot}{Cl}}{:} + \cdot\overset{\displaystyle\cdot\cdot}{\underset{\displaystyle\cdot\cdot}{Cl}}{:} \rightarrow {:}\overset{\displaystyle\cdot\cdot}{\underset{\displaystyle\cdot\cdot}{Cl}}{:}\overset{\displaystyle\cdot\cdot}{\underset{\displaystyle\cdot\cdot}{Cl}}{:}$$

Covalent bonds are the most plentiful type of bond making up the human body. They are typically found in molecules containing carbon. Only six elements typically form covalent bonds: carbon (C), nitrogen (N), phosphorus (P), oxygen (O), sulfur (S), and hydrogen (H). Covalent bonds are a crucial source of energy for living organisms. Covalent bonds are comparable in strength to ionic bonds, but stronger than hydrogen bonds, and are typically used to bind the basic macromolecules—carbohydrates, lipids, nucleic acids, and proteins—together.

Hydrogen Bonding

Hydrogen bonds are temporary and weak. They typically occur between two partial, opposite electrical charges. For example, hydrogen bonds form when a hydrogen (H) atom in the vicinity of nitrogen (N), fluorine (F), or oxygen (O) atoms. These partial electrical charges are called *dipoles,* and are caused by the unequal sharing of electrons between covalent bonds. Water is the most prevalent molecule that forms hydrogen bonds.

Hydrogen bonds contribute to the adhesiveness and cohesiveness properties of molecules like water. Adhesiveness confers glue-like properties to molecules which ensure they stick or connect more easily with other molecules, similar to wetting a suction cup before sticking it to a surface. Cohesiveness refers to a molecule's ability to form hydrogen bonds with itself. For example, the cohesiveness of water is the reason why it has a high boiling point, which is a physical property.

Metallic Bonds

Metallic bonds are formed by electrons that move freely through the metal. They are the product of the force of attraction between electrons and metal ions. The electrons are shared by many metal cations and act like a glue holding the metallic substance together, similar to the attraction between oppositely charged atoms in ionic substances except the electrons are more fluid and float around the bonded metals and form a "sea of electrons". Metallic compounds have characteristic properties including strength, conduction of heat and electricity, and malleability. They can conduct electricity by passing energy through the freely moving electrons, creating a current. These compounds also have high melting and boiling points. Lewis structures are not common for metallic structures because of the free-roaming ability of the electrons.

Explaining Characteristic Properties of Substances

Properties of Water

Water is the most abundant substance on Earth. It is a compound composed of hydrogen and oxygen with the chemical formula H_2O. Water is also *polar*, which means it is negatively charged at one end and positively charged at the other end. The oxygen is more *electronegative* than the hydrogens, meaning that its protons pull in more of the electrons than do the hydrogens. This leaves the oxygen with a partial negative charge and the hydrogens with a partial positive charge.

Water is *amphoteric* and *self-ionizable* in that it tends to dissociate, or split, into hydrogen ions (H^+) and hydroxyl ions (OH^-) randomly. No other substance on Earth may be found naturally in all three states of matter—liquid, solid, and gas. Water is also unique due to it liquid state being more dense than its solid state (ice), which is why ice floats in liquid water. Water is colorless, odorless, and tasteless. It freezes at 32 ^0F and boils at 212 ^0F. Pure water has a pH of 7, which makes it neutral. Water is considered the universal solvent because it can dissolve many substances.

Many of the properties of water are due to its polarity and hydrogen bonding. Water has the following properties:

- Cohesiveness: Refers to the force of attraction between molecules of identical substances. Cohesiveness is mainly the result of hydrogen bonding in water.

- Adhesiveness: Refers to the force of attraction between molecules of different substances. For example, water and glass. Adhesiveness is mainly the result of hydrogen bonding in water.

- High specific heat: Refers to the amount of heat required to raise the temperature of water by one degree Celsius. Water's high specific heat is a consequence of hydrogen bonding. As a result, water can store a great deal of heat energy.

- High surface tension: The cohesiveness of water molecules is responsible for its high surface tension. The strong cohesion of its molecules makes water sticky and elastic.

- High heat of vaporization: Refers to the energy required to transform a given amount of water from a liquid to a gas at a given pressure. Water's high heat of vaporization is due to hydrogen bonding.

Characteristic Properties of Molecules

Molecules have both physical and chemical properties. Physical properties describe a substance in isolation, while chemical properties describe how a substance reacts with others.

There are two types of physical properties: extensive and intensive. Extensive physical properties depend on the amount of a substance. Volume, length, and mass are all examples of extensive properties.

Intensive physical properties are static and unchanging properties of a substance that identify it. Examples of intensive physical properties include the following:

- Color
- Smell
- Taste
- Odor
- Luster: Ability to reflect light, also known as "shininess"
- Hardness: Ability to scratch
- Brittleness: Response to pressure. The more brittle, the easier it is to break.
- Malleability: Ability to bend
- Ductility: Ability to form wire
- Conductivity: Ability to conduct heat and electricity
- Polarity: Extent to which a covalent molecule has a partial charge due to the unequal sharing of electrons
- Melting Point
- Boiling Point
- Density (mass/volume)

Extensive properties are important for measurement and recording data, but do not identify a substance. Intensive properties are critical for identification, as indicated by the following examples.

You find a brittle, yellow, dull rock that smells like rotten eggs. *What is it?* All signs point to sulfur; however, pure sulfur has no smell so it has to be some sort of sulfur mixture.

You buy a beautiful ring and are unsure if it is silver, white gold, or platinum. They all have the same color, are shiny, and conduct heat. *So which metal is it?* To find the difference, more information would be needed. Platinum is much harder than gold and not easily scratched. Silver is significantly less dense than the other two. By examining the physical properties and comparing them to the physical properties of silver, white gold, and platinum, determining its composition should be no problem.

Physical changes do not change the intensive physical properties of a substance. For example, cutting paper into pieces will not change its density, hardness, or luster. Shattering glass does not change the physical properties either; it is still clear and not malleable or ductile. Pouring water into a differently shaped container won't change its melting or boiling points.

Chemical changes, on the other hand, transform substances so that they have new physical properties. For example, upon exposing iron to air it will form a completely different substance. The product of iron and oxygen is rust, a reddish substance.

While physical properties describe the characteristics of a substance, chemical like properties describe how it *behaves* in chemical reactions.

- If substances are flammable, they burn easily in chemical reactions.
- If substances are radioactive, they emit radiation in nuclear reactions.
- If substances are corrosive, they are capable of degrading or eating away other substances.
- If substances are easily oxidized, they will react quickly with air.

Comparing and Contrasting Changes in States of Matter

States of Matter—Liquids, Gases, and Solids
There are three fundamental states of matter—liquid, gas, and solid. The molecules in a liquid are not in an orderly arrangement and can move past one another. Weak intermolecular forces contribute to a liquid having an indefinite shape, but definite volume. Lastly, a liquid conforms to the shape of its container, is not easily compressible, and flows quite easily.

The molecules in a gas have a large amount of space between them. A gas will diffuse indefinitely if unconfined, while it will assume the shape and volume of its container if enclosed. In other words, a gas has no definite shape or volume. Lastly, a gas is compressible and flows quite easily.

The molecules in a solid are closely packed together, which restricts their movement. Very strong intermolecular forces contribute to a solid having a definite shape and volume. Furthermore, a solid is not easily compressible and does not flow easily.

Vaporization, Evaporation, and Condensation
States of matter are able to undergo phase transitions. Vaporization refers to the transformation of a solid or liquid into a gas. There are two types of vaporization—evaporation and boiling. Evaporation is a surface phenomenon and involves the conversion of a liquid into a gas below the boiling temperature at a given pressure. Evaporation is also an important component of the water cycle. Boiling occurs below the surface and involves the conversion of liquid into a gas at or above the boiling temperature. Condensation represents the conversion of a gas into a liquid. It is the reverse of evaporation. Condensation is also most often synonymous with the water cycle. It is a crucial component of distillation.

Phase Transitions

Matter exists in phases and is mostly in the solid, liquid, or gas form. Solid matter has particles packed closely together. Solids are not compressible because they are already so compact that they are actually vibrating due to the significant attractive and repulsive intermolecular forces. Solids have no flow and do not take the shape of their container. Liquids, on the other hand, have flow because particles are not as tightly packed. They take the shape of their container but are not easily compressible because the particles are still fairly close together. Gas particles are different from solids and liquids in that they are very easily compressible. They are so far apart that intermolecular forces are negligible.

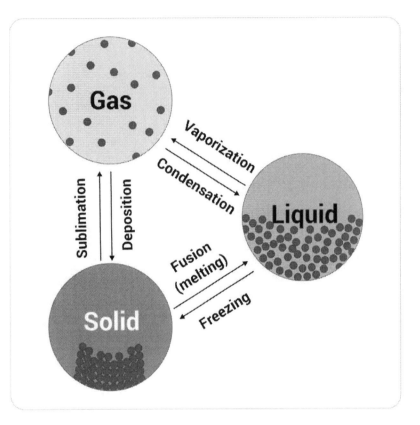

Phase changes are best described in terms of temperature and kinetic energy. Consider a tightly packed solid that has particles very close together. If heat is added, kinetic energy of the molecules increase. If enough heat is added, the particles will move quickly enough that they will begin to slide past each other and form a liquid. Moving from a solid to a liquid is called *melting*. The opposite change is *freezing*. Freezing occurs when liquid particles move slower and pack closely together into a solid.

Think of liquid water heating on a stove. When the boiling point is reached, some of the particles will turn into gas because they have so much kinetic energy. Moving from this liquid from into a gas is called *vaporization*. The opposite reaction is *condensation* which occurs when gas particles slow down and form a liquid. This is seen on the exterior of a cold drink when water vapor in the air cools on the glass and forms water beads.

Less common are direct changes from either solid to gas, or *sublimation*, or from a gas to a solid, or *deposition*. Sublimation appears as a solid emitting a cloud, like dry ice. Deposition can happen with water in extremely cold temperatures. Frost is water that has gone directly from a gas to a solid.

Describing Chemical Reactions

<u>Types of Chemical Reactions</u>
Chemical reactions are characterized by a chemical change in which the starting substances, or reactants, differ from the substances formed, or products. Chemical reactions may involve a change in color, the production of gas, the formation of a precipitate, or changes in heat content. The following are the five basic types of chemical reactions:

Reaction Type	Definition	Example
Decomposition	A compound is broken down into two or more smaller elements or compounds.	$2H_2O \rightarrow 2H_2 + O_2$
Synthesis	Two or more elements or compounds are joined together.	$2H_2 + O_2 \rightarrow 2H_2O$
Single Displacement	A single element or ion takes the place of another in a compound. Also known as a substitution reaction.	$Zn + 2HCl \rightarrow ZnCl_2 + H_2$
Double Displacement	Two elements or ions exchange a single atom each to form two different compounds, resulting in different combinations of cations and anions in the final compounds. Also known as a metathesis reaction.	$H_2SO_4 + 2NaOH \rightarrow Na_2So_4 + 2H_2O$
Oxidation-Reduction	Elements undergo a change in oxidation number. Also known as a redox reaction.	$2S_2O_3^{2-}(aq) + I_2(aq) \rightarrow S_4O_6^{2-}(aq) + 2I^-$ (aq)
Acid-Base	Involves a reaction between an acid and a base, which usually produces a salt and water	$HBr + NaOH \rightarrow NaBr + H_2O$
Combustion	A hydrocarbon (a compound composed of only hydrogen and carbon) reacts with oxygen to form carbon dioxide and water.	$CH_4 + 2O_2 \rightarrow CO_2 + 2H_2O$

<u>Balancing Chemical Reactions</u>
Chemical reactions are expressed using chemical equations. Chemical equations must be balanced with equivalent numbers of atoms for each type of element on each side of the equation. Antoine Lavoisier, a French chemist, was the first to propose the Law of Conservation of Mass for the purpose of balancing a chemical equation. The law states, "Matter is neither created nor destroyed during a chemical reaction."

The reactants are located on the left side of the arrow, while the products are located on the right side of the arrow. Coefficients are the numbers in front of the chemical formulas. Subscripts are the numbers to the lower right of chemical symbols in a formula. To tally atoms, one should multiply the formula's coefficient by the subscript of each chemical symbol. For example, the chemical equation $2 H_2 + O_2 \rightarrow 2H_2O$ is balanced. For H, the coefficient of 2 multiplied by the subscript 2 = 4 hydrogen atoms. For O, the coefficient of 1 multiplied by the subscript 2 = 2 oxygen atoms. Coefficients and subscripts of 1 are understood and never written. When known, the form of the substance is noted with (g)=gas, (s)=solid, (l)=liquid, or (aq)=aqueous.

Catalysts

Catalysts are substances that accelerate the speed of a chemical reaction. A catalyst remains unchanged throughout the course of a chemical reaction. In most cases, only small amounts of a catalyst are needed. Catalysts increase the rate of a chemical reaction by providing an alternate path requiring less activation energy. Activation energy refers to the amount of energy required for the initiation of a chemical reaction.

Catalysts can be homogeneous or heterogeneous. Catalysts in the same phase of matter as its reactants are homogeneous, while catalysts in a different phase than reactants are heterogeneous. It is important to remember catalysts are selective. They don't accelerate the speed of all chemical reactions, but catalysts do accelerate specific chemical reactions.

Enzymes

Enzymes are a class of catalysts instrumental in biochemical reactions, and in most, if not all, instances are proteins. Like all catalysts, enzymes increase the rate of a chemical reaction by providing an alternate path requiring less activation energy. Enzymes catalyze thousands of chemical reactions in the human body. Enzymes are proteins and possess an active site, which is the part of the molecule that binds the reacting molecule, or substrate. The "lock and key" analogy is used to describe the substrate key fitting precisely into the active site of the enzyme lock to form an enzyme-substrate complex.

Many enzymes work in tandem with cofactors or coenzymes to catalyze chemical reactions. *Cofactors* can be either inorganic (not containing carbon) or organic (containing carbon). Organic cofactors can be either coenzymes or prosthetic groups tightly bound to an enzyme. *Coenzymes* transport chemical groups from one enzyme to another. Within a cell, coenzymes are continuously regenerating and their concentrations are held at a steady state.

Several factors including temperature, pH, and concentrations of the enzyme and substrate can affect the catalytic activity of an enzyme. For humans, the optimal temperature for peak enzyme activity is approximately body temperature at 98.6 ^{0}F, while the optimal pH for peak enzyme activity is approximately 7-8. Increasing the concentrations of either the enzyme or substrate will also increase the rate of reaction, up to a certain point.

The activity of enzymes can be regulated. One common type of enzyme regulation is termed *feedback inhibition*, which involves the product of the pathway inhibiting the catalytic activity of the enzyme involved in its manufacture.

pH, Acids, and Bases
pH refers to the power or potential of hydrogen atoms and is used as a scale for a substance's acidity. In chemistry, pH represents the hydrogen ion concentration (written as [H^+]) in an aqueous, or watery, solution. The hydrogen ion concentration, [H^+], is measured in moles of H^+ per liter of solution.

The pH scale is a logarithmic scale used to quantify how acidic or basic a substance is. pH is the negative logarithm of the hydrogen ion concentration: pH = -log [H^+]. A one-unit change in pH correlates with a ten-fold change in hydrogen ion concentration. The pH scale typically ranges from 0 to 14, although it is possible to have pHs outside of this range. Pure water has a pH of 7, which is considered neutral. pH values less than 7 are considered acidic, while pH values greater than 7 are considered basic, or alkaline.

Generally speaking, an acid is a substance capable of donating hydrogen ions, while a base is a substance capable of accepting hydrogen ions. A buffer is a molecule that can act as either a hydrogen ion donor or acceptor. Buffers are crucial in the blood and body fluids, and prevent the body's pH from fluctuating into dangerous territory. pH can be measured using a pH meter, test paper, or indicator sticks.

Protons, Neutrons, and Electrons

The structure of an atom has two major components: the atomic nucleus and the atomic shells. The nucleus is found in the center of an atom. The three major subatomic particles are protons, neutrons, and electrons and are found in the atomic nucleus and shells.

Protons are found in the atomic nucleus and are positively charged particles. The addition or removal of protons from an atom's nucleus creates an entirely different element. *Neutrons* are also found in the atomic nucleus and are neutral particles, meaning they have no net electrical charge. The addition or removal of neutrons from an atom's nucleus does not create a different element but instead creates a lighter or heavier form of that element called an isotope. *Electrons* are found orbiting in the atomic shells around the nucleus and are negatively charged particles. A proton or a neutron has nearly 2,000 times the mass of an electron.

Electrons and Chemical Bonds

Electrons orbit the nucleus in atomic shells. For example, the first atomic shell can accommodate two electrons, the second atomic shell can hold a maximum of eight electrons, and the third atomic shell can house a maximum of eight electrons. The negatively charged electrons orbiting the nucleus are attracted to the positively charged protons in the nucleus via electromagnetic force. The attraction of opposite electrical charges gives rise to chemical bonds, which refers to the ways atoms are attached to each other.

Chemical bonding typically results in the formation of a new substance. Only the electrons in the outermost atomic shell are able to form chemical bonds. These electrons are known as valence electrons, and they are what determines the chemical properties of an atom.

Chemical Bonds Between Atoms

Chemical bonds refer to the manner in which atoms are attached to one another. Atoms may be held together with three fundamental types of chemical bonds—ionic, covalent, or hydrogen.

Ionic Bonding

In an *ionic bond*, an atom loses one or more electrons to another who gains them. The atoms do this so that they can achieve a full outermost shell of electrons, which is the configuration with the lowest amount of energy, and these are typically the strongest types of bonds. Ionic bonds typically occur metals and nonmetals to form salts like $MgCl_2$ and BF_3. When an atom has a different number of electrons than its number of protons, it is termed an *ion*. A positively charged ion is referred to as a *cation*, while a negatively charged ion is referred to as an *anion*. For example, a sodium cation (Na^{+1}) can form an ionic bond to a chlorine anion (Cl^{-1}) to form sodium chloride (NaCl), which is also known as table salt. The majority of the molecules formed with ionic bonds such as this have a crystalline structure.

Covalent Bonding

In a *covalent bond*, two or more atoms share one or more electrons. Covalent bonds are the most plentiful type of bond making up the human body. They are typically found in molecules containing carbon. Only six elements typically form covalent bonds: carbon (C), nitrogen (N), phosphorus (P), oxygen (O), sulfur (S), and hydrogen (H). Covalent bonds are a crucial source of energy for living organisms. Covalent bonds are comparable in strength to ionic bonds, but stronger than hydrogen bonds, and are typically used to bind the basic macromolecules—carbohydrates, lipids, nucleic acids, and proteins—together.

Hydrogen Bonding

Hydrogen bonds are temporary and weak. They typically occur between two partial, opposite electrical charges. For example, hydrogen bonds form when a hydrogen (H) atom in the vicinity of nitrogen (N), fluorine (F), or oxygen (O) atoms. These partial electrical charges are called *dipoles,* and are caused by the unequal sharing of electrons between covalent bonds. Water is the most prevalent molecule that forms hydrogen bonds.

Hydrogen bonds contribute to the adhesiveness and cohesiveness properties of molecules like water. Adhesiveness confers glue-like properties to molecules which ensure they stick or connect more easily with other molecules, similar to wetting a suction cup before sticking it to a surface. Cohesiveness refers to a molecule's ability to form hydrogen bonds with itself. For example, the cohesiveness of water is the reason why it has a high boiling point, which is a physical property.

Scientific Reasoning

Identifying Basic Scientific Measurement Using Laboratory Tools

Technology and mathematics are crucial to the advancement of scientific investigations and communications. Individuals in specialized scientific fields need answers to problems swiftly, as they are frequently under time constraints. Accurate and prompt scientific investigation is dependent on technological and mathematical skills and their advancement. Advances in technology and mathematics can help accelerate the pace of scientific investigations and communications.

Although scientific investigations can be communicated to some degree through subjective qualitative data, objective quantitative data is preferred to establish rigorous mathematical conclusions. Connections can also be conveyed through the use of graphs, formulas, and equations. Mathematical relationships can be proven with numerical models.

Software like spreadsheets and networks like the Internet have expanded scientific communication by providing multiple avenues to distribute information. Increased computing capacity and fiber optics have also increased the speed and processing time of scientific communication.

Reasons for Including Technology and Mathematics in Science Research
There are many different reasons for including technology and mathematics in science research. Technology is always advancing and its application is playing an increasingly larger role in science research. Technology enhances the gathering and manipulation of scientific data. Technology also increases the accuracy and precision of scientific data, which in many ways is becoming more dependent on the type of technology adopted. Graphs or models can be produced to highlight emerging patterns or trends in scientific data which can be used to improve the interpretation and understanding of specific scientific data from the past or present.

Mathematics has been around for centuries and has constantly been called upon in scientific research to help understand and explain the workings of the natural world. It is a crucial part of the scientific method. Mathematics can help improve and refine the asking of questions or hypotheses in a scientific argument. Advances in mathematics have led to improvements in gathering data, constructing scientific explanations, and communicating results of scientific investigations. Lastly, mathematics has improved the efficiency of processing and manipulating often complicated scientific data.

When recording data, it is of the utmost importance to also record units. Acceptable customary units in the U.S. include feet, gallon, and pound which measure length, volume, and mass, respectively. Laboratory data is typically recorded with SI units which are universally used. Standard SI units include the following:

- Second (s) for time
- Meter (m) for length
- Gram (g) for mass
- Liter (L) for volume
- Celsius (^{o}C) $-$ or $-$ Kelvin (K) for temperature (^{o}C + 273 = K)

Prefixes also indicate the scale, as seen in the chart below.

Other important concepts regarding collecting data are scientific notation, rounding, and significant figures.

Scientific notation should be used when appropriate. The correct form is to have the ones unit followed by the decimal point with the appropriate amount of significant figures followed by an indication of the power of ten.

$1,320,000 = 1.32 \times 10^6$

$0.000867 = 8.67 \times 10^{-4}$

Rounding should be used to the correct number of significant figures. 0-4 always keeps the preceding number as is while 5-9 raises it.

1.325 rounds to 1.33

4.289 rounds to 1.29

5.998 rounds to 6.00

Significant figures should be used, meaning that measurements too precise to be recorded should not be included. This concept is illustrated in the following scenarios.

A balance that goes to the hundredths place measures a rock as 1.92. It would be incorrect to record the value as 2 or 1.9 (remember rounding rules) because that is not precise enough. It would also be incorrect to record the value as 1.920 because that implies a level of precision that does not exist with that measuring device.

Examine the three rulers below and the line being measured. While the length of the line remains the same, the different calibrations of the rulers result in answers with a different number of significant figures. The top ruler cannot even give a level of certainty to the ones place so the appropriate number of significant figures is 1. The middle ruler does have a calibration that allows a measurement to the ones place so there are two significant figures. The bottom ruler can record a reading with 3 significant figures.

Measuring volume with a graduated cylinder is tricky because the liquid will look curved. The curve, or meniscus, is due to the adhesion of the water to the sides of the device. The bottom of the meniscus indicates the actual volume of the liquid. In this case, recording the value as 35 would be incorrect. The calibration of the graduated cylinder calls for a greater level of precision in any data taken, and the data recorded needs to reflect that. The correct value is 35.0.

Significant figures have a few rules. Any non-zero number preceding a decimal point is significant and any trailing zeros are not significant. Zeroes between numbers are always significant. After the decimal point, any preceding zeroes are not significant while any trailing zeroes are.

- 3,570,000 has 3 significant figures.
- 4, 000, 560 has 6 significant figures.
- 0.000008320 has 4 significant figures.
- 0.00903 has 3 significant figures.

<u>Scale</u>
Different situations call for different units of measurement, or different scales. It is important to be mindful of scale especially when working in medicine. Anesthesia administration is weight-dependent, so it is critical to make sure that the weight is correctly labeled as either kilograms or pounds.

Kilograms or pounds, on the other hand, are inappropriate measurements for very small objects. Chemists and physicists do calculations with atoms and molecules which require a completely different unit. They use a unit called the mole which contains 6.02×10^{23} particles of a substance.

Temperature has three different scales: Kelvin, Celsius, and Fahrenheit. Kelvin is required for gas calculations, and should engineers use the wrong conversion, gas tanks could explode or be completely non-functional.

Critiquing a Scientific Explanation Using Logic and Evidence

A scientific explanation has three crucial components—a claim, evidence, and logical reasoning. A claim makes an assertion or conclusion focusing on the original question or problem. The evidence provides backing for the claim and is usually in the form of scientific data. The scientific data must be appropriate and sufficient. The scientific reasoning connects the claim and evidence and explains why the evidence supports the claim.

Scientific explanations must fit certain criteria and be supported by logic and evidence. The following represent scientific explanation criteria. The proposed explanation:

- Must be logically consistent
- Must abide by the rules of evidence
- Must report procedures and methods
- Must be open to questions and possible modification
- Must be based on historical and current scientific knowledge

The scientific method encourages the growth and communication of new information and procedures among scientists. Explanations of how the natural world shifts based on fiction, personal convictions, religious morals, mystical influences, superstitions, or authorities are not scientific and therefore irrelevant.

Scientific explanations have two fundamental characteristics. First, they should explain all scientific data and observations gleaned from experiments. Second, they should allow for predictions that can be verified with future experiments.

It's important to focus on the *empirical*, or observable/tangible evidence, in an experiment. After all, an experiment is about testing something, not theorizing about it in the abstract. Doing so helps remove a researcher's personal *bias* towards what they think or hope to be true.

Explaining Relationships Among Events, Objects, and Processes

<u>Cause and Effect</u>
A cause is like a stimulus in the nervous system in that it results in a response. An effect is what happens because of the stimulus.

Cause	Effect
I forgot to wear shoes.	I stubbed my toe.
I forgot to practice piano.	I messed up at the recital and was embarrassed.
I studied for my math exam.	I got a 100.

The cause is the *why* something happens, and the effect is what actually happens.

While it is typical for there to be a single cause and a single effect as noted above, there are many situations that call for a cause to have many effects, such as exploring the effects of a certain event. In exploring the effects of exercise, for example, the cause is exercise. Effects are stress relief, increased energy, and weight loss.

There is the possibility that one effect can have many causes. For example, type 2 diabetes is not a one-cause disease, but rather a combination of exercise habits, diet, and genetics.

A cause-and-effect chain is when an effect then causes another effect. For example, the initial cause could be when a young gentleman played video games instead of studying for a biology test, which sets off a chain reaction of effects.

- 1st effect: He failed the test.
- 2nd effect: He got in trouble with his parents.
- 3rd effect: He couldn't hang out with his friends on Friday night.
- 4th effect: He had a boring night.
-

<u>Unit Size</u>
In understanding relationships between objects encountered in science (such as parts of the human body), it's important to roughly understand the scale of them. This is accomplished by understanding the size of different units of measurement and knowing which unit makes the most sense for measuring something.
For example, you could record the distances between cities in centimeters but miles or kilometers makes the most sense. Be sure the memorize the metric prefixes discussed in the math section. That will give you an indication of how big or small a unit is.

Analyzing the Design of a Scientific Investigation

The scientific method provides the framework for studying and learning about the world in a scientific fashion. The scientific method has been around since at least the 17th century and is a codified way to answer natural science questions. Due to objectivity, the scientific method is impartial and its results are highly repeatable; these are its greatest advantages.

There is no consensus as to the number of steps involved in executing the scientific method, but the following six steps are needed to fulfill the criteria for correct usage of the scientific method:

- Ask a question: Most scientific investigations begin with a question about a specific problem.

- Make observations: Observations will help pinpoint research objectives on the quest to answer the question.

- Create or propose a hypothesis: The hypothesis represents a possible solution to the problem. It is a simple statement predicting the outcome of an experiment testing the hypothesis.

- Formulate an experiment: The experiment tests the proposed hypothesis.

- Test the hypothesis: The outcome of the experiment to test the hypothesis is the most crucial step in the scientific method.

- Accept or reject the hypothesis: Using results from the experiment, a scientist can conclude to accept or reject the hypothesis.

Several key nuances of the scientific method include:

- The hypothesis must be verifiable and falsifiable. Falsifiable refers to the possibility of a negative solution to the hypothesis. The hypothesis should also have relevance, compatibility, testability, simplicity, and predictive power.

- Investigation must utilize both deductive and inductive reasoning. Deductive reasoning employs a logical process to arrive at a conclusion using premises considered true, while inductive reasoning employs an opposite approach. Inductive reasoning allows scientist to propose hypotheses in the scientific method, while deductive reasoning allows scientist to apply hypotheses to particular situations.

- An experiment should incorporate an independent, or changing, variable and a dependent, or non-changing, variable. It should also utilize both a control group and an experimental group. The experimental group will ultimately be compared against the control group.

Practice Questions

1. Which statement about white blood cells is true?
    a. B cells are responsible for antibody production.
    b. White blood cells are made in the white/yellow cartilage before they enter the bloodstream.
    c. Platelets, a special class of white blood cell, function to clot blood and stop bleeding.
    d. The majority of white blood cells only activate during the age of puberty, which explains why children and the elderly are particularly susceptible to disease.

2. Which locations in the digestive system are sites of chemical digestion?
    I. Mouth
    II. Stomach
    III. Small Intestine

    a. II only
    b. III only
    c. II and III only
    d. I, II, and III

4. Which of the following structures is unique to eukaryotic cells?
    a. Cell walls
    b. Nucleuses
    c. Cell membranes
    d. Vacuoles

5. Which is the cellular organelle used for digestion to recycle materials?
    a. The Golgi apparatus
    b. The lysosome
    c. The centrioles
    d. The mitochondria

6. A rock has a mass of 14.3 grams (g) and a volume of 5.4 cm^3, what is its density?
    a. 8.90 g/cm^3
    b. 0.38 g/cm^3
    c. 77.22 g/cm^3
    d. 2.65 g/cm^3

7. Why do arteries have valves?
    a. They have valves to maintain high blood pressure so that capillaries diffuse nutrients properly.
    b. Their valves are designed to prevent backflow due to their low blood pressure.
    c. They have valves due to a leftover trait from evolution that, like the appendix, are useless.
    d. They do not have valves, but veins do.

8. If the pressure in the pulmonary artery is increased above normal, which chamber of the heart will be affected first?
    a. The right atrium
    b. The left atrium
    c. The right ventricle
    d. The left ventricle

9. What is the purpose of sodium bicarbonate when released into the lumen of the small intestine?
    a. It works to chemically digest fats in the chyme.
    b. It decreases the pH of the chyme so as to prevent harm to the intestine.
    c. It works to chemically digest proteins in the chyme.
    d. It increases the pH of the chyme so as to prevent harm to the intestine.

10. Which of the following describes a reflex arc?
    a. The storage and recall of memory
    b. The maintenance of visual and auditory acuity
    c. The autoregulation of heart rate and blood pressure
    d. A stimulus and response controlled by the spinal cord

11. Describe the synthesis of the lagging strand of DNA.
    a. DNA polymerases synthesize DNA continuously after initially attaching to a primase.
    b. DNA polymerases synthesize DNA discontinuously in pieces called Okazaki fragments after initially attaching to primases.
    c. DNA polymerases synthesize DNA discontinuously in pieces called Okazaki fragments after initially attaching to RNA primers.
    d. DNA polymerases synthesize DNA discontinuously in pieces called Okazaki fragments which are joined together in the end by a DNA helicase.

12. Using anatomical terms, what is the relationship of the sternum relative to the deltoid?
    a. Medial
    b. Lateral
    c. Superficial
    d. Posterior

13. Ligaments connect what?
    a. Muscle to muscle
    b. Bone to bone
    c. Bone to muscle
    d. Muscle to tendon

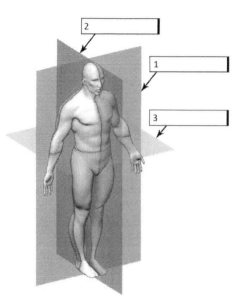

14. Identify the correct sequence of the 3 primary body planes as numbered 1, 2, and 3 in the above image.
    a. Plane 1 is coronal, plane 2 is sagittal, and plane 3 is transverse.
    b. Plane 1 is sagittal, plane 2 is coronal, and plane 3 is medial.
    c. Plane 1 is coronal, plane 2 is sagittal, and plane 3 is medial.
    d. Plane 1 is sagittal, plane 2 is coronal, and plane 3 is transverse.

15. Which of the following is NOT a major function of the respiratory system in humans?
    a. It provides a large surface area for gas exchange of oxygen and carbon dioxide.
    b. It helps regulate the blood's pH.
    c. It helps cushion the heart against jarring motions.
    d. It is responsible for vocalization.

16. Which of the following is NOT a function of the forebrain?
    a. To regulate blood pressure and heart rate
    b. To perceive and interpret emotional responses like fear and anger
    c. To perceive and interpret visual input from the eyes
    d. To integrate voluntary movement

17. What is the major difference between somatic and germline mutations?
    a. Somatic mutations usually benefit the individual while germline mutations usually harm them.
    b. Since germline mutations only affect one cell, they are less noticeable than the rapidly dividing somatic cells.
    c. Somatic mutations are not expressed for several generations, but germline mutations are expressed immediately.
    d. Germline mutations are usually inherited while somatic mutations will affect only the individual.

18. A child complains of heavy breathing even when relaxing. They are an otherwise healthy child with no history of respiratory problems. What might be the issue?
    a. Asthma
    b. Blood clot
    c. Hyperventilation
    d. Exercising too hard

19. Find the lowest coefficients that will balance the following combustion equation.

$$\_\_C_2H_{10}+\_\_O_2 \rightarrow \_\_H_2O+\_\_CO_2$$

    a. 1:5:5:2
    b. 4:10:20:8
    c. 2:9:10:4
    d. 2:5:10:4

20. What is the purpose of a catalyst?
    a. To increase a reaction rate by increasing the activation energy
    b. To increase a reaction's rate by increasing the temperature
    c. To increase a reaction's rate by decreasing the activation energy
    d. To increase a reaction's rate by decreasing the temperature

21. Most catalysts found in biological systems are which of the following?
    a. Special lipids called cofactors.
    b. Special proteins called enzymes.
    c. Special lipids called enzymes.
    d. Special proteins called cofactors.

22. Which statement is true about the pH of a solution?
    a. A solution cannot have a pH less than 1.
    b. The more hydroxide ions in the solution, the higher the pH.
    c. If an acid has a pH of greater than 2, it is considered a weak base.
    d. A solution with a pH of 2 has ten times the amount of hydrogen ions than a solution with a power of 1.

23. Salts like sodium iodide (NaI) and potassium chloride (KCl) use what type of bond?
    a. Ionic bonds
    b. Disulfide bridges
    c. Covalent bonds
    d. London dispersion forces

24. Which of the following is unique to covalent bonds?
    a. Most covalent bonds are formed between the elements H, F, N, and O.
    b. Covalent bonds are dependent on forming dipoles.
    c. Bonding electrons are shared between two or more atoms.
    d. Molecules with covalent bonds tend to have a crystalline solid structure.

25. Which of the following describes a typical gas?
    a. Indefinite shape and indefinite volume
    b. Indefinite shape and definite volume
    c. Definite shape and definite volume
    d. Definite shape and indefinite volume

26. Which of the following areas of the body has the most sweat glands?
    a. Upper back
    b. Arms
    c. Feet
    d. Palms

27. A patient's body is not properly filtering blood. Which of the following body parts is most likely malfunctioning?
    a. Medulla
    B. Heart
    C. Nephrons
    D. Renal cortex

28. A pediatrician notes that an infant's cartilage is disappearing and being replaced by bone. What process has the doctor observed?
    a. Mineralization
    b. Ossification
    c. Osteoporosis
    d. Calcification

29. The epidermis is compose of what type of cells?
    a. Osteoclasts
    b. Connective
    c. Dendritic
    d. Epithelial

30. Which of the following is directly transcribed from DNA and represents the first step in protein building?
    a. siRNA
    b. rRNA
    c. mRNA
    d. tRNA

31. What information does a genotype give that a phenotype does not?
    a. The genotype necessarily includes the proteins coded for by its alleles.
    b. The genotype will always show an organism's recessive alleles.
    c. The genotype must include the organism's physical characteristics.
    d. The genotype shows what an organism's parents looked like.

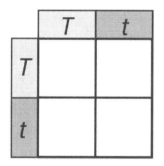

32. Which statement is supported by the Punnett square above, if "T" = Tall and "t" = short?
    a. Both parents are homozygous tall.
    b. 100% of the offspring will be tall because both parents are tall.
    c. There is a 25% chance that an offspring will be short.
    d. The short allele will soon die out.

33. Which of the following is a chief difference between evaporation and boiling?
   a. Liquids boil only at the surface while they evaporate equally throughout the liquid.
   b. Evaporating substances change from gas to liquid while boiling substances change from liquid to gas.
   c. Evaporation happens in nature while boiling is a manmade phenomenon.
   d. Evaporation can happen below a liquid's boiling point.

34. Which of the following CANNOT be found in a human cell's genes?
   a. Sequences of amino acids to be transcribed into mRNA
   b. Lethal recessive traits like sickle cell anemia
   c. Mutated DNA
   d. DNA that codes for proteins the cell doesn't use

35. Which of the following is a special property of water?
   a. Water easily flows through phospholipid bilayers.
   b. A water molecule's oxygen atom allows fish to breathe.
   c. Water is highly cohesive which explains its high melting point.
   d. Water can self-hydrolyze and decompose into hydrogen and oxygen.

36. What is an isotope? For any given element, it is an atom with which of the following?
   a. a different atomic number.
   b. a different number of protons.
   c. a different number of electrons.
   d. a different mass number.

37. What is the electrical charge of the nucleus?
   a. A nucleus always has a positive charge.
   b. A stable nucleus has a positive charge, but a radioactive nucleus may have no charge and instead be neutral.
   c. A nucleus always has no charge and is instead neutral.
   d. A stable nucleus has no charge and is instead neutral, but a radioactive nucleus may have a charge.

38. A student believes that there is an inverse relationship between sugar consumption and test scores. To test this hypothesis, he recruits several people to eat sugar, wait one hour, and take a short aptitude test afterwards. The student will compile the participants' sugar intake levels and test scores. How should the student conduct the experiment?
   a. One round of testing, where each participant consumes a different level of sugar.
   b. Two rounds of testing: The first, where each participant consumes a different level of sugar, and the second, where each participant consumes the same level as they did in Round 1.
   c. Two rounds of testing: The first, where each participant consumes the same level of sugar as each other, and the second, where each participant consumes the same level of sugar as each other but at higher levels than in Round 1.
   d. One round of testing, where each participant consumes the same level of sugar.

39. Which of the following creates sperm?
   a. Prostate gland
   b. Seminal vesicles
   c. Scrotum
   d. Seminiferous tubules

40. A researcher is exploring factors that contribute to the GPA of college students. While the sample is small, the researcher is trying to determine what the data shows. What can be reasoned from the table below?

Student	Maintains a Calendar?	Takes Notes?	GPA
A	sometimes	often	3.1
B	never	always	3.9
C	never	never	2.0
D	sometimes	often	2.7

a. No college students consistently maintain a calendar of events.

b. There is an inverse correlation between maintaining a calendar and GPA, and there is a positive correlation between taking notes and GPA.

c. There is a positive correlation between maintaining a calendar and GPA, and there is no correlation between taking notes and GPA.

d. There is no correlation between maintaining a calendar and GPA, and there is a positive correlation between taking notes and GPA.

41. Four different groups of the same species of peas are grown and exposed to differing levels of sunlight, water, and fertilizer as documented in the table below. The data in the water and fertilizer columns indicates how many times the peas are watered or fertilized per week, respectively. Group 2 is the only group that withered. What is a reasonable explanation for this occurrence?

Group	Sunlight	Water	Fertilizer
1	partial sun	4 mL/hr	1
2	full sun	7 mL/hr	1
3	no sun	14 mL/hr	2
4	partial sun	3 mL/hr	2

a. Insects gnawed away the stem of the plant.

b. The roots rotted due to poor drainage.

c. The soil type had nutrition deficiencies.

d. This species of peas does not thrive in full sunlight.

42. Which of the following functions corresponds to the parasympathetic nervous system?
   a. It stimulates the fight-or-flight response.
   b. It increases heart rate.
   c. It stimulates digestion.
   d. It increases bronchiole dilation.

43. According to the periodic table, which of the following elements is the least reactive?
   a. Fluorine
   b. Silicon
   c. Neon
   d. Gallium

44. The Human Genome Project is a worldwide research project launched in 1990 to map the entire human genome. Although the Project was faced with the monumental challenge of analyzing tons and tons of data, its objective was completed in 2003 and ahead of its deadline by two years. Which of the following inventions likely had the greatest impact on this project?

    a. The sonogram

    b. X-ray diffraction

    c. The microprocessor

    d. Magnetic Resonance Imaging (MRI)

45. Which of the following inventions likely had the greatest improvement on the ability to combat nutrition deficiencies in developing countries?

    a. Food products fortified with dietary vitamins and minerals

    b. Integrated statistical models of fish populations

    c. Advances so that microscopes can use thicker tissue samples

    d. Refrigerated train cars for transportation of food

46. Which of the following is the gland that helps regulate calcium levels?

    a. Osteotoid gland

    b. Pineal gland

    c. Parathyroid glands

    d. Thymus gland

47. Anya was paid by Company X to analyze dwindling honeybee populations of the Southwest. After measuring hive populations over several months, she noticed no patterns in the geographic distributions of the deaths after comparisons with local maps of interest. This supported her hypothesis, so she took samples of the honey and the bees from the hives and performed dozens of dissections to confirm her suspicions. Which of the following is the most likely hypothesis upon which this research was performed?

    a. Honeybees are being killed off and their hives destroyed by other extremely aggressive species of bees from the South.

    b. Honeybees are contracting parasites in large droves.

    c. Honeybees are so sensitive to certain pesticides that they die on contact.

    d. Honeybees die in larger numbers around cell phone towers.

48. Explain the Law of Conservation of Mass as it applies to this reaction: $2H_2 + O_2 \rightarrow 2H_2O$.

    a. Electrons are lost.

    b. The hydrogen loses mass.

    c. New oxygen atoms are formed.

    d. There is no decrease or increase of matter

49. Which of the following is the best unit to measure the amount of blood in the human body?

    a. Ounces

    b. Liters

    c. Milliliters

    d. Pounds

50. Which of the following systems does not include a transportation system throughout the body?

    a. Cardiovascular system

    b. Endocrine system

    c. Immune system

    d. Nervous system

51. Which of the following correctly identifies a difference between the primary and secondary immune response?

a. In the secondary response, macrophages migrate to the lymph nodes to present the foreign microorganism to helped T lymphocytes.

b. The humeral immunity that characterizes the primary response is coordinated by T lymphocytes.

c. The primary response is quicker and more powerful than the secondary response.

d. Suppressor T cells activate in the secondary response to prevent an overactive immune response.

52. Eosinophils are best described as which of the following?

a. A type of granulocyte that secretes histamine, which stimulates the inflammatory response.

b. The most abundant type of white blood cell and they secrete substances that are toxic to pathogens.

c. A type of granulocyte found under mucous membranes and defends against multicellular parasites.

d. A type of circulating granulocyte that is aggressive and has high phagocytic activity.

53. Which of the following correctly matches a category of protein with a physiologic example?

a. Keratin is a structural protein

b. Antigens are hormonal proteins

c. Channel proteins are marker proteins

d. Actin is a transport protein

Answer Explanations

1. A: When activated, B cells create antibodies against specific antigens. White blood cells are generated in yellow bone marrow, not cartilage. Platelets are not a type of white blood cell, and are typically cell fragments produced by megakaryocytes. White blood cells are active throughout nearly all of one's life, and have not been shown to specially activate or deactivate because of life events like puberty or menopause.

2. D: Mechanical digestion is physical digestion of food and tearing it into smaller pieces using force. This occurs in the stomach and mouth. Chemical digestion involves chemically changing the food and breaking it down into small organic compounds that can be utilized by the cell to build molecules. The salivary glands in the mouth secrete amylase that breaks down starch, which begins chemical digestion. The stomach contains enzymes such as pepsinogen/pepsin and gastric lipase, which chemically digest protein and fats, respectively. The small intestine continues to digest protein using the enzymes trypsin and chymotrypsin. It also digests fats with the help of bile from the liver and lipase from the pancreas. These organs act as exocrine glands because they secrete substances through a duct. Carbohydrates are digested in the small intestine with the help of pancreatic amylase, gut bacterial flora and fauna, and brush border enzymes like lactose. Brush border enzymes are contained in the towel-like microvilli in the small intestine that soak up nutrients.

4. B: The structure exclusively found in eukaryotic cells is the nucleus. Animal, plant, fungi, and protist cells are all eukaryotic. DNA is contained within the nucleus of eukaryotic cells, and they also have membrane-bound organelles that perform complex intracellular metabolic activities. Prokaryotic cells (archae and bacteria) do not have a nucleus or other membrane-bound organelles and are less complex than eukaryotic cells.

5. B: The cell structure responsible for cellular storage, digestion and waste removal is the lysosome. Lysosomes are like recycle bins. They are filled with digestive enzymes that facilitate catabolic reactions to regenerate monomers. The Golgi apparatus is designed to tag, package, and ship out proteins destined for other cells or locations. The centrioles typically play a large role only in cell division when they ratchet the chromosomes from the mitotic plate to the poles of the cell. The mitochondria are involved in energy production and are the powerhouses of the cell.

6. D: Density is found by dividing mass by volume:

$$density = \frac{mass}{volume}$$

The unit for mass (in this case grams) and the units for volume (in this case cm^3) need to be combined together. They're combined as grams over volume since that's how they were set up in the equation:

$$d = \frac{14.3\ g}{5.4\ cm^3} = 2.65\ g/cm^3$$

7. D: Veins have valves, but arteries do not. Valves in veins are designed to prevent backflow, since they are the furthest blood vessels from the pumping action of the heart and steadily increase in volume (which decreases the available pressure). Capillaries diffuse nutrients properly because of their thin walls and high surface area and are not particularly dependent on positive pressure.

8. C: The blood leaves the right ventricle through a semi-lunar valve and goes through the pulmonary artery to the lungs. Any increase in pressure in the artery will eventually affect the contractibility of the right ventricle. Blood enters the right atrium from the superior and inferior venae cava veins, and blood leaves the right atrium through the tricuspid valve to the right ventricle. Blood enters the left atrium from the pulmonary veins carrying oxygenated blood from the lungs. Blood flows from the left atrium to the left ventricle through the mitral valve and leaves the left ventricle through a semi-lunar valve to enter the aorta.

9. D: Sodium bicarbonate, a very effective base, has the chief function to increase the pH of the chyme. Chyme leaving the stomach has a very low pH, due to the high amounts of acid that are used to digest and break down food. If this is not neutralized, the walls of the small intestine will be damaged and may form ulcers. Sodium bicarb is produced by the pancreas and released in response to pyloric stimulation so that it can neutralize the acid. It has little to no digestive effect.

10. D: A reflex arc is a simple nerve pathway involving a stimulus, a synapse, and a response that is controlled by the spinal cord—not the brain. The knee-jerk reflex is an example of a reflex arc. The stimulus is the hammer touching the tendon, reaching the synapse in the spinal cord by an afferent pathway. The response is the resulting muscle contraction reaching the muscle by an efferent pathway. None of the remaining processes is a simple reflex. Memories are processed and stored in the hippocampus in the limbic system. The visual center is located in the occipital lobe, while auditory processing occurs in the temporal lobe. The sympathetic and parasympathetic divisions of the autonomic nervous system control heart and blood pressure.

11. C: The lagging strand of DNA falls behind the leading strand because of its discontinuous synthesis. DNA helicase unzips the DNA helices so that synthesis can take place, and RNA primers are created by the RNA primase for the polymerases to attach to and build from. The lagging strand is synthesizing DNA in a direction that is hard for the polymerase to build, so multiple primers are laid down so that the entire length of DNA can be synthesized simultaneously, piecemeal. These short pieces of DNA being synthesized are known as Okazaki fragments and are joined together by DNA ligase.

12. A: The sternum is medial to the deltoid because it is much closer (typically right on) the midline of the body, while the deltoid is lateral at the shoulder cap. Superficial means that a structure is closer to the body surface and posterior means that it falls behind something else. For example, skin is superficial to bone and the kidneys are posterior to the rectus abdominus.

13. B: Ligaments connect bone to bone. Tendons connect muscle to bone. Both are made of dense, fibrous connective tissue (primary Type 1 collagen) to give strength. However, tendons are more organized, especially in the long axis direction like muscle fibers themselves, and they have more collagen. This arrangement makes more sense because muscles have specific orientations of their fibers, so they contract in somewhat predictable directions. Ligaments are less organized and more of a woven pattern because bone connections are not as organized as bundles or muscle fibers, so ligaments must have strength in multiple directions to protect against injury.

14. A: The three primary body planes are coronal, sagittal, and transverse. The coronal or frontal plane, named for the plane in which a corona or halo might appear in old paintings, divides the body vertically into front and back sections. The sagittal plane, named for the path an arrow might take when shot at the body, divides the body vertically into right and left sections. The transverse plane divides the body horizontally into upper or superior and lower or inferior sections. There is no medial plane, per se. The anatomical direction medial simply references a location close or closer to the center of the body than another location.

15. C: Although the lungs may provide some cushioning for the heart when the body is violently struck, this is not a major function of the respiratory system. Its most notable function is that of gas exchange for oxygen and carbon dioxide, but it also plays a vital role in the regulation of blood pH. The aqueous form of carbon dioxide, carbonic acid, is a major pH buffer of the blood, and the respiratory system directly controls how much carbon dioxide stays and is released from the blood through respiration. The respiratory system also enables vocalization and forms the basis for the mode of speech and language used by most humans.

16. A: The forebrain contains the cerebrum, the thalamus, the hypothalamus, and the limbic system. The limbic system is chiefly responsible for the perception of emotions through the amygdale, while the cerebrum interprets sensory input and generates movement. Specifically, the occipital lobe receives visual input, and the primary motor cortex in the frontal lobe is the controller of voluntary movement. The hindbrain, specifically the medulla oblongata and brain stem, control and regulate blood pressure and heart rate.

17. D: Germline mutations in eggs and sperm are permanent, can be on the chromosomal level, and will be inherited by offspring. Somatic mutations cannot affect eggs and sperm, and therefore are not inherited by offspring. Mutations of either kind are rarely beneficial to the individual, but do not necessarily harm them. Germline cells divide much more rapidly than do somatic cells, and a mutation in a sex cell would promulgate and affect many thousands of its daughter cells.

18. A: It is most likely asthma. Any of the answer choices listed can cause heavy breathing. A blood clot in the lung (*B*) could cause this, but this would be very uncommon for a child. Choices *C* and *D* can both be ruled out because the question mentions that it occurs even when the patient is relaxing. Hyperventilation is usually caused by a panic attack or some sort of physical activity. Asthma often develops during childhood. It would stand to reason then that the child may have not yet been diagnosed. While asthma attacks can be caused by exercise they can also occur when a person is not exerting themselves.

19. C: 2:9:10:4. These are the coefficients that follow the law of conservation of matter. The coefficient times the subscript of each element should be the same on both sides of the equation.

20. C: A catalyst functions to increase reaction rates by decreasing the activation energy required for a reaction to take place. Inhibitors would increase the activation energy or otherwise stop the reactants from reacting. Although increasing the temperature usually increases a reaction's rate, this is not true in all cases, and most catalysts do not function in this manner.

21. B: Biological catalysts are termed *enzymes*, which are proteins with conformations that specifically manipulate reactants into positions which decrease the reaction's activation energy. Lipids do not usually affect reactions, and cofactors, while they can aid or be necessary to the proper functioning of enzymes, do not make up the majority of biological catalysts.

22. B: Substances with higher amounts of hydrogen ions will have lower pHs, while substances with higher amounts of hydroxide ions will have higher pHs. Choice *A* is incorrect because it is possible to have an extremely strong acid with a pH less than 1, as long as its molarity of hydrogen ions is greater than 1. Choice *C* is false because a weak base is determined by having a pH lower than some value, not higher. Substances with pHs greater than 2 include anything from neutral water to extremely caustic lye. Choice *D* is false because a solution with a pH of 2 has ten times fewer hydrogen ions than a solution of pH 1.

23. A: Salts are formed from compounds that use ionic bonds. Disulfide bridges are special bonds in protein synthesis which hold the protein in their secondary and tertiary structures. Covalent bonds are strong bonds formed through the sharing of electrons between atoms and are typically found in organic molecules like carbohydrates and lipids. London dispersion forces are fleeting, momentary bonds which occur between atoms that have instantaneous dipoles but quickly disintegrate.

24. C: As in the last question, covalent bonds are special because they share electrons between multiple atoms. Most covalent bonds are formed between the elements H, F, N, O, S, and C, while hydrogen bonds are formed nearly exclusively between H and either O, N, or F. Covalent bonds may inadvertently form dipoles, but this does not necessarily happen. With similarly electronegative atoms like carbon and hydrogen, dipoles do not form, for instance. Crystal solids are typically formed by substances with ionic bonds like the salts sodium iodide and potassium chloride.

25. A: Gases like air will move and expand to fill their container, so they are considered to have an indefinite shape and indefinite volume. Liquids like water will move and flow freely, so their shapes change constantly, but do not change volume or density on their own. Solids change neither shape nor volume without external forces acting on them, so they have definite shapes and volumes.

26. A: The upper back has the one of the high densities of sweat glands of any area on the body. While palms, arms, and feet are often thought of as sweaty areas, they have relatively low amounts of sweat glands compared to other parts of the body. Remember that one of the purposes of sweat is thermoregulation, or controlling the temperature of the body. Regulating the temperature of one's core is more important than adjusting the temperature of one's extremities.

27. C: Nephrons are responsible for filtering blood. When functioning properly they allow blood cells and nutrients to go back into the bloodstream while sending waste to the bladder. However, nephrons can fail at doing this, particularly when blood flood to the kidneys is limited. The medulla (also called the renal medulla) (*A*) and the renal cortex (*D*) are both parts of the kidney but are not specifically responsible for filtering blood. The medulla is in the inner part of the kidney and contains the nephrons. The renal cortex is the outer part of the kidney. The heart (*B*) is responsible for pumping blood throughout the body rather than filtering it.

28. B: Ossification is the process by which cartilage, a soft, flexible substance is replaced by bone throughout the body. All humans regardless of age have cartilage, but cartilage in some areas goes away to make way for bones.

29. D: The outermost layer of the skin, the epidermis, consists of epithelial cells. This layer of skin is dead, as it has no blood vessels. Osteoclasts are cells that make up bones. Notice the prefix *Osteo-* which means bone. Connective tissue macrophage cells can be found in a variety of places, and dendritic cells are part of the lymphatic system.

30. C: mRNA is directly transcribed from DNA before being taken to the cytoplasm and translated by rRNA into a protein. tRNA transfers amino acids from the cytoplasm to the rRNA for use in building these proteins. siRNA is a special type of RNA which interferes with other strands of mRNA typically by causing them to get degraded by the cell rather than translated into protein.

31. B: Since the genotype is a depiction of the specific alleles that an organism's genes code for, it includes recessive genes that may or may not be otherwise expressed. The genotype does not have to name the proteins that its alleles code for; indeed, some of them may be unknown. The phenotype is the physical, visual manifestations of a gene, not the genotype. The genotype does not necessarily include any information about the organism's physical characters. Although some information about an organism's parents can be obtained from its genotype, its genotype does not actually show the parents' phenotypes.

32. C: One in four offspring (or 25%) will be short, so all four offspring cannot be tall. Although both of the parents are tall, they are hybrid or heterozygous tall, not homozygous. The mother's phenotype is for tall, not short. A Punnett square cannot determine if a short allele will die out. Although it may seem intuitive that the short allele will be expressed by lower numbers of the population than the tall allele, it still appears in 75% of the offspring (although its effects are masked in 2/3 of those). Besides, conditions could favor the recessive allele and kill off the tall offspring.

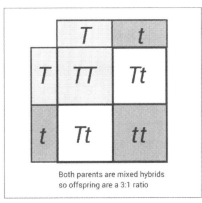

Both parents are mixed hybrids
so offspring are a 3:1 ratio

33. D: Evaporation takes place at the surface of a fluid while boiling takes place throughout the fluid. The liquid will boil when it reaches its boiling or vaporization temperature, but evaporation can happen due to a liquid's volatility. Volatile substances often coexist as a liquid and as a gas, depending on the pressure forced on them. The phase change from gas to liquid is condensation, and both evaporation and boiling take place in nature.

34. A: Human genes are strictly DNA and do not include proteins or amino acids. A human's genome and collection of genes will include even their recessive traits, mutations, and unused DNA.

35. C: Water's polarity lends it to be extremely cohesive and adhesive; this cohesion keeps its atoms very close together. Because of this, it takes a large amount of energy to melt and boil its solid and liquid forms. Phospholipid bilayers are made of nonpolar lipids and water, a polar liquid, cannot flow through it. Cell membranes use proteins called aquaporins to solve this issue and let water flow in and out. Fish breathe by capturing dissolved oxygen through their gills. Water can self-ionize, wherein it decomposes into a hydrogen ion (H^+) and a hydroxide ion (OH^-), but it cannot self-hydrolyze.

36. D: An isotope of an element has an atomic number equal to its number of protons, but a different mass number because of the additional neutrons. Even though there are differences in the nucleus, the behavior and properties of isotopes of a given element are identical. Atoms with different atomic numbers also have different numbers of protons and are different elements, so they cannot be isotopes.

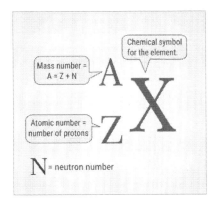

Chemical symbol for the element.

Mass number = $A = Z + N$

Atomic number = number of protons

N = neutron number

195

37. A: The neutrons and protons make up the nucleus of the atom. The nucleus is positively charged due to the presence of the protons. The negatively charged electrons are attracted to the positively charged nucleus by the electrostatic or Coulomb force; however, the electrons are not contained in the nucleus. The positively charged protons create the positive charge in the nucleus, and the neutrons are electrically neutral, so they have no effect. Radioactivity does not directly have a bearing on the charge of the nucleus.

38. C: To gather accurate data, the student must be able compare a participant's test score from round 1 with their test score from round 2. The differing levels of intellect among the participants means that comparing participants' test scores to those of other participants would be inaccurate. This requirement excludes choices A and D, which involve only one round of testing. The experiment must also involve different levels of sugar consumption from round 1 to round 2. In this way, the effects of different levels of sugar consumption can be seen on the same subjects. Thus, B is incorrect because the experiment provides for no variation of sugar consumption. C is the correct answer because it allows the student to compare each participant's test score from round 1 with their test score from round 2 after different level of sugar consumption.

39. D: The seminiferous tubules are responsible for sperm production. Had *testicles* been an answer choice, it would also have been correct since it houses the seminiferous tubules. The prostate gland (*A*) secretes enzymes that help nourish sperm after creation. The seminal vesciles (*B*) secrete some of the components of semen. The scrotum (*C)* is the pouch holding the testicles.

40. D: Based on this table, it can be reasoned that there is not a correlation between maintaining a calendar and GPA, since Student B never maintains a calendar but has the highest GPA of the cohort. Furthermore, it can be reasoned that there is a positive correlation between taking notes and GPA since the more notes a student takes, the higher the GPA that they have. Thus, Choice *D* is the correct answer. Choice *A* offers an absolute that cannot be proven based on this study; thus, it is incorrect. Choices B and C are incorrect because they have at least one incorrect correlation.

41. D: *D* is the correct answer because excess sunlight is a common cause of plant wilting. *A, B,* and *C* are all possible but unlikely to be a cause for wilting. Given that the test question asks for a *reasonable* explanation, *sunlight* is by far the most reasonable answer.

42. C: The parasympathetic nervous system is related to calm, peaceful times without stress that require no immediate decisions. It relaxes the fight-or-flight response, slows heart rate to a comfortable pace, and decreases bronchiole dilation to a normal size. The sympathetic nervous system, on the other hand, is in charge of the fight-or-flight response and works to increase blood pressure and oxygen absorption.

43. C: Neon, one of the noble gases, is chemically inert or not reactive because it contains eight valence electrons in the outermost shell. The atomic number is 10, with a 2.8 electron arrangement meaning that there are 2 electrons in the inner shell and the remaining 8 electrons in the outer shell. This is extremely stable for the atom, so it will not want to add or subtract any of its electrons and will not react under typical circumstances.

44. C: Because of the vast amounts of data that needed to be processed and analyzed, technological breakthroughs like innovations to the microprocessor were directly responsible for the ease of computing handled by the Human Genome Project. Although the sonogram and MRI technology are helpful to the healthcare industry in general, they would not have provided a great deal of help for sequencing and comprehending DNA data, in general. X-ray diffraction is a technique that helps visualize the structures of crystallized proteins, but cannot determine DNA bases with enough precision to help sequence DNA.

45. A: Many foods from developed countries are grown from plants which have been processed or bioengineered to include increased amounts of nutrients like vitamins and minerals that otherwise would be lost during manufacturing or are uncommon to the human diet. White rice, for example, is typically enriched with niacin, iron, and folic acid, while salt has been fortified with iodine for nearly a century. These help to prevent nutrition deficiencies. While it can be useful for fisheries to maintain models of fish populations so that they don't overfish their stock, this is not as immediately important to nutrition as are fortified and enriched foods. Although innovations to microscopes could lead to improved healthcare, this also has no direct effect on nutrition deficiency. Refrigerated train carts were historically a crucial invention around Civil War times and were used to transport meat and dairy products long distances without spoiling, but dietary deficiencies could be more easily remedied by supplying people with fortified foods containing those nutrients rather than spoilable meats.

46. C: The parathryroid gland impacts calcium levels by secreting parathyroid hormone (PTH). Osteotoid gland is not a real gland. The pineal gland regulates sleep by secreting melatonin, and the thymus gland focuses on immunity. *Thyroid* would also be a correct answer choice as it influences the levels of circulating calcium.

47. B: The most likely hypothesis that Anya is testing has something to with the pathophysiology of the bees, as she performed dissections on some of her samples. These dissections would be unnecessary if the bees were being killed off by another species, as the destruction of the hives would be obvious. As the deaths did not seem linked in any particular way geographically, it is also safe to assume that there was no correlation to cell phone towers, as maps of cell phone coverage would be readily available to her. If the pesticides were so toxic that the bees died on contact, then they wouldn't make it back to the hive to be available for her dissections or to drop off chemicals in the honey. The most likely of the choices is that parasites are killing off the bees, which would be easily communicable.

48. D: The law states that matter cannot be created or destroyed in a closed system. In this equation, there are the same number of molecules of each element on either side of the equation. Matter is not gained or lost, although a new compound is formed. As there are no ions on either side of the equation, no electrons are lost. The law prevents the hydrogen from losing mass and prevents oxygen atoms from being spontaneously spawned.

49. B: For measuring blood, we're looking for a unit that measures volume. Choices *A, B,* and *C,* are all measures of volume, but pounds (*D*) is a measure of weight. The correct answer is liters, as the average adult has about 5 liters of blood in their body. Blood can certainly be measured in ounces or milliliters; however, 5 liters is equal to 5,000 milliliters or 176 ounces. Thus, liters seems to be the more rational measuring unit.

50. B: The endocrine system's organs are glands which are spread throughout the body. The endocrine system itself does not connect the organs or transport the hormones they secrete. Rather, the various glands secrete the hormone into the bloodstream and lets the cardiovascular system pump it throughout the body. The other three body systems each include a network throughout the body:

- Cardiovascular system: veins and arteries
- Immune system: lymphatic vessels (it does also use the circulatory system)
- Nervous system: nerve networks

51. D: In the secondary immune response, suppressor T lymphocytes are activated to negate the potential risk of damage to healthy cells, brought on by an unchecked, overactive immune response. Choice *A* is incorrect because the activity is characteristic of the primary response, not the secondary response Choice *B* is incorrect because humeral immunity is mediated by antibodies produced by B, not T, lymphocytes. Choice *C* is wrong because the secondary response is faster than the primary response because the primary response entails the time-consuming process of macrophage activation.

52. C: Eosinophils, like neutrophils, basophils, and mast cells, are a type of leukocyte in a class called granulocytes. They are found underneath mucous membranes in the body and they primarily secrete destructive enzymes and defend against multicellular parasites like worms. Choice *A* describes basophils and mast cells, and Choice *B* and *D* describe neutrophils. Unlike neutrophils which are aggressive phagocytic cells, eosinophils have low phagocytic activity.

53. A: Keratin is a structural protein and it is the primary constituent of things like hair and nails. Choice *B* is incorrect antigens are immune proteins that help fight disease. Hormonal proteins are responsible for initiating the signal transduction cascade to regulate gene expression. Choice *C* is incorrect because channel proteins are transport proteins that help move molecules into and out of a cell. Marker proteins help identify or distinguish a cell. Lastly, Choice *D* is incorrect because actin, like myosin, is a motor protein because it is involved in the process of muscle contraction.

English and Language Usage

Conventions of Standard English

Conventions of Standard English Spelling

Spelling might or might not be important to some, or maybe it just doesn't come naturally, but those who are willing to discover some new ideas and consider their benefits can learn to spell better and improve their writing. Misspellings reduce a writer's credibility and can create misunderstandings. Spell checkers built into word processors are not a substitute for accuracy. They are neither foolproof nor without error. In addition, a writer's misspelling of one word may also be a word. For example, a writer intending to spell *herd* might accidentally type *s* instead of *d* and unintentionally spell *hers*. Since *hers* is a word, it would not be marked as a misspelling by a spell checker. In short, use spell check, but don't rely on it.

Guidelines for Spelling

Saying and listening to a word serves as the beginning of knowing how to spell it. Keep these subsequent guidelines in mind, remembering there are often exceptions because the English language is replete with them.

Guideline #1: Syllables must have at least one vowel. In fact, every syllable in every English word has a vowel.

- d*o*g
- h*a*yst*a*ck
- *a*nsw*e*r*i*ng
- *a*bst*e*nt*iou*s
- s*i*mpl*e*

Guideline #2: The long and short of it. When the vowel has a short vowel sound as in *mad* or *bed,* only the single vowel is needed. If the word has a long vowel sound, add another vowel, either alongside it or separated by a consonant: bed/*bead*; mad/*made.* When the second vowel is separated by two spaces— *madder*—it does not affect the first vowel's sound.

Guideline #3: Suffixes. Refer to the examples listed above.

Guideline #4: Which comes first; the *i* or the *e*? Remember the saying, "*I* before *e* except after *c* or when sounding as *a* as in *neighbor* or *weigh.*" Keep in mind that these are only guidelines and that there are always exceptions to every rule.

Guideline #5: Vowels in the right order. Another helpful rhyme is, "When two vowels go walking, the first one does the talking." When two vowels are in a row, the first one often has a long vowel sound and the other is silent. An example is *team.*

If you have difficulty spelling words, determine a strategy to help. Work on spelling by playing word games like Scrabble or Words with Friends. Consider using phonics, which is sounding words out by slowly and surely stating each syllable. Try repeating and memorizing spellings as well as picturing words in your head. Try making up silly memory aids. See what works best.

Homophones

Homophones are two or more words that have no particular relationship to one another except their identical pronunciations. Homophones make spelling English words fun and challenging like these:

Common Homophones		
affect, effect	cell, sell	it's, its
allot, a lot	do, due, dew	knew, new
barbecue, barbeque	dual, duel	libel, liable
bite, byte	eminent, imminent	principal, principle
brake, break	flew, flu, flue	their, there, they're
capital, capitol	gauge, gage	to, too, two
cash, cache	holy, wholly	yoke, yolk

Irregular Plurals

Irregular plurals are words that aren't made plural the usual way.

- Most nouns are made plural by adding *–s* (book*s*, television*s*, skyscraper*s*).

- Most nouns ending in *ch, sh, s, x,* or *z* are made plural by adding *–es* (church*es*, marsh*es*).

- Most nouns ending in a vowel + *y* are made plural by adding *–s* (day*s*, toy*s*).

- Most nouns ending in a consonant + *y,* are made plural by the *-y* becoming *-ies* (baby becomes *babies*).

- Most nouns ending in an *o* are made plural by adding *–s* (piano*s*, photo*s*).

- Some nouns ending in an *o,* though, may be made plural by adding *–es* (example: potato*es,* volcano*es*), and, of note, there is no known rhyme or reason for this!

- Most nouns ending in an *f* or *fe* are made plural by the *-f* or *-fe* becoming *-ves*! (example: wolf becomes *wolves*).

- Some words function as both the singular and plural form of the word (fish, deer).

- Other exceptions include *man* becomes *men, mouse* becomes *mice, goose* becomes *geese,* and *foot* becomes *feet.*

Contractions

The basic rule for making *contractions* is one area of spelling that is pretty straightforward: combine the two words by inserting an apostrophe (') in the space where a letter is omitted. For example, to combine *you* and *are,* drop the *a* and put the apostrophe in its place: *you're.*

> he + is = he's
> you + all = y'all (informal but often misspelled)

Note that *it's,* when spelled with an apostrophe, is always the contraction for *it is.* The possessive form of the word is written without an apostrophe as *its.*

Correcting Misspelled Words

A good place to start looking at commonly misspelled words here is with the word *misspelled*. While it looks peculiar, look at it this way: *mis* (the prefix meaning *wrongly*) + *spelled* = *misspelled*.

Let's look at some commonly misspelled words and see where writers often go wrong with them.

Commonly Misspelled Words					
accept	benign	existence	jewelry	parallel	separate
acceptable	bicycle	experience	judgment	pastime	sergeant
accidentally	brief	extraordinary	library	permissible	similar
accommodate	business	familiar	license	perseverance	supersede
accompany	calendar	February	maintenance	personnel	surprise
acknowledgement	campaign	fiery	maneuver	persuade	symmetry
acquaintance	candidate	finally	mathematics	possess	temperature
acquire	category	forehead	mattress	precede	tragedy
address	cemetery	foreign	millennium	prevalent	transferred
aesthetic	changeable	foremost	miniature	privilege	truly
aisle	committee	forfeit	mischievous	pronunciation	usage
altogether	conceive	glamorous	misspell	protein	valuable
amateur	congratulations	government	mortgage	publicly	vengeance
apparent	courtesy	grateful	necessary	questionnaire	villain
appropriate	deceive	handkerchief	neither	recede	Wednesday
arctic	desperate	harass	nickel	receive	weird
asphalt	discipline	hygiene	niece	recommend	
associate	disappoint	hypocrisy	ninety	referral	
attendance	dissatisfied	ignorance	noticeable	relevant	
auxiliary	eligible	incredible	obedience	restaurant	
available	embarrass	intelligence	occasion	rhetoric	
balloon	especially	intercede	occurrence	rhythm	
believe	exaggerate	interest	omitted	schedule	
beneficial	exceed	irresistible	operate	sentence	

Capitalization

Here's a non-exhaustive list of things that should be capitalized.

- the first word of every sentence
- the first word of every line of poetry
- the first letter of proper nouns (World War II)
- holidays (Valentine's Day)
- days of the week and months of the year (Tuesday, March)
- the first word, last word, and all major words in the titles of books, movies, songs, and other creative works (*To Kill a Mockingbird,* note that *a* is lowercase since it's not a major word, but *to* is capitalized since it's the first word of the title.
- titles when preceding a proper noun (President Roberto Gonzales, Aunt Judy)

When simply using a word such as president or secretary, though, the word is not capitalized.

> Officers of the new business must include a *president* and *treasurer*.

Seasons—spring, fall, etc.—are not capitalized.

North, south, east, and *west* are capitalized when referring to regions but are not when being used for directions. In general, if it's preceded by *the* it should be capitalized.

> I'm from the South.
> I drove south.

Conventions of Standard English Punctuation

Ellipses
An *ellipsis* (...) consists of three handy little dots that can speak volumes on behalf of irrelevant material. Writers use them in place of a word(s), line, phrase, list contents, or paragraph that might just as easily have been omitted from a passage of writing. This can be done to save space or to focus only on the specifically relevant material.

> Exercise is good for some unexpected reasons. Watkins writes, "Exercise has many benefits such as ...reducing cancer risk."

In the example above, the ellipsis takes the place of the other benefits of exercise that are more expected.

The ellipsis may also be used to show a pause in sentence flow.

> "I'm wondering...how this could happen," Dylan said in a soft voice.

Commas
A *comma* (,) is the punctuation mark that signifies a pause—breath—between parts of a sentence. It denotes a break of flow. As with so many aspects of writing structure, authors will benefit by reading their writing aloud or mouthing the words. This can be particularly helpful if one is uncertain about whether the comma is needed.

In a complex sentence—one that contains a subordinate (dependent) clause or clauses—separate the clauses with commas.

> I will not pay for the steak, *because I don't have that much money.*

First, see how the purpose of each comma usage is to designate an interruption in flow. Then, notice how the last clause is dependent because it requires the earlier independent clauses to make sense.

Use a comma on both sides of an interrupting phrase.

> I will pay for the ice cream, *chocolate and vanilla,* and I will eat it all myself.

The words forming the phrase in italics are nonessential (extra) information. To determine if a phrase is nonessential, try reading the sentence without the phrase and see if it's still coherent.

A comma is not necessary in this next sentence because no interruption—nonessential or extra information— has occurred. Read sentences aloud when uncertain.

I will pay for his chocolate and vanilla ice cream and I will eat it all myself.

If the nonessential phrase comes at the beginning of a sentence, a comma should only go at the end of the phrase. If the phrase comes at the end of a sentence, a comma should only go at the beginning of the phrase.

Other types of interruptions include the following:

- interjections: Oh no, I am not going.
- abbreviations: Barry Potter, M.D., specializes in heart disorders.
- direct addresses: Yes, Claudia, I am tired and going to bed.
- parenthetical phrases: His wife, lovely as she was, was not helpful.
- transitional phrases: Also, it is not possible.

The second comma in the following sentence is called an Oxford comma.

I will pay for ice cream, syrup, and pop.

It is a comma used after the second-to-last item in a series of three or more items. It comes before the word *or* or *and*. Not everyone uses the Oxford comma; it is optional, but many believe it is needed. The comma functions as a tool to reduce confusion in writing. So, if omitting the Oxford comma would cause confusion, then it's best to include it.

Commas are used in math to mark the place of thousands in numerals, breaking them up so they are easier to read. Other uses for commas are in dates (*March 19, 2016*), letter greetings (*Dear Sally,*), and in between cities and states (*Louisville, KY*).

Semicolons
The *semicolon* (;) might be described as a heavy-handed comma. Take a look at these two examples:

I will pay for the ice cream and I will pay for the syrup, but I will not pay for the steak.
I will pay for the ice cream and I will pay for the syrup; I will not pay for the steak.

What's the difference? The first example has a comma and a conjunction separating the two independent clauses. The second example does not have a conjunction, but there are two independent clauses in the sentence. So something more than a comma is required. In this case, a semicolon is used.

Two independent clauses can only be joined in a sentence by either a comma and conjunction or a semicolon. If one of those tools is not used, the sentence will be a run-on. Remember that while the clauses are independent, they need to be closely related in order to be contained in one sentence.

Another use for the semicolon is to separate items in a list when the items themselves require commas.

The family lived in Phoenix, Arizona; Oklahoma City, Oklahoma; and Raleigh, North Carolina.

Colons
Colons have many miscellaneous functions. Colons can be used to proceed further information or a list. In these cases, a colon should only follow an independent clause.

Humans take in sensory information through five basic senses: sight, hearing, smell, touch, and taste.

The meal includes the following components:

- Caesar salad
- spaghetti

- garlic bread
- cake

The family got what they needed: a reliable vehicle.

While a comma is more common, a colon can also proceed a formal quotation.

> He said to the crowd: "Let's begin!"

The colon is used after the greeting in a formal letter.

> Dear Sir:
> To Whom It May Concern:

In the writing of time, the colon separates the minutes from the hour (*4:45 p.m.*). The colon can also be used to indicate a ratio between two numbers (*50:1*).

Hyphens

The *hyphen* (-) is a little hash mark that can be used to join words to show that they are linked.

Hyphenate two words that work together as a single adjective (a compound adjective).

> honey-covered biscuits

Some words always require hyphens, even if not serving as an adjective.

> merry-go-round

Hyphens always go after certain prefixes like *anti-* & *all-*.

Hyphens should also be used when the absence of the hyphen would cause a strange vowel combination (*semi-engineer*) or confusion. For example, *re-collect* should be used to describe something being gathered twice rather than being written as *recollect*, which means to remember.

Parentheses and Dashes

Parentheses are half-round brackets that look like this: ( ). They set off a word, phrase, or sentence that is a afterthought, explanation, or side note relevant to the surrounding text but not essential. A pair of commas is often used to set off this sort of information, but parentheses are generally used for information that would not fit well within a sentence or that the writer deems not important enough to be structurally part of the sentence.

> The picture of the heart (see above) shows the major parts you should memorize.
> Mount Everest is one of three mountains in the world that are over 28,000 feet high (K2 and Kanchenjunga are the other two).

See how the sentences above are complete without the parenthetical statements? In the first example, *see above* would not have fit well within the flow of the sentence. The second parenthetical statement could have been a separate sentence, but the writer deemed the information not pertinent to the topic.

The dash (—) is a mark longer than a hyphen used as a punctuation mark in sentences and to set apart a relevant thought. Even after plucking out the line separated by the dash marks, the sentence will be intact and make sense.

> Looking out the airplane window at the landmarks—Lake Clarke, Thompson Community College, and the bridge—she couldn't help but feel excited to be home.

The dashes use is similar to that of parentheses or a pair of commas. So, what's the difference? Many believe that using dashes makes the clause within them stand out while using parentheses is subtler. It's advised to not use dashes when commas could be used instead.

Quotation Marks

The uses of quotation marks was discussed under the category *Dialogue.* Other uses include:

- around titles of songs, short stories, essays, and chapter in books
- to emphasize a certain word
- to refer to a word as the word itself
- Example: What's the meaning of *indubitably*?

Apostrophes

This punctuation mark, the apostrophe (') is a versatile little mark. It has a few different functions:

- Quotes: Apostrophes are used when a second quote is needed within a quote.

- In my letter to my friend, I wrote, "The girl had to get a new purse, and guess what Mary did? She said, 'I'd like to go with you to the store.' I knew Mary would buy it for her."

- Contractions: Another use for an apostrophe in the quote above is a contraction. *I'd* is used for *I would.*

- Possession: An apostrophe followed by the letter *s* shows possession (*Mary's* purse). If the possessive word is plural, the apostrophe generally just follows the word.

- The trees' leaves are all over the ground.

Various Sentence Structures

Sentence Fluency

It's time to take what's been studied and put it all together in order to construct well-written sentences and paragraphs that have correct structure. Learning and utilizing the mechanics of structure will encourage effective, professional results, and adding some creativity will elevate one's writing to a higher level.

First, let's review the basic elements of sentences.

A *sentence* is a set of words that make up a grammatical unit. The words must have certain elements and be spoken or written in a specific order to constitute a complete sentence that makes sense.

> 1. A sentence must have a *subject* (a noun or noun phrase). The subject tells whom or what the sentence is addressing (i.e. what it is about).

> 2. A sentence must have an *action* or *state of being* (*a verb*). To reiterate: A verb forms the main part of the predicate of a sentence. This means that it explains what the noun is doing.

3. A sentence must convey a complete thought.

When examining writing, be mindful of grammar, structure, spelling, and patterns. Sentences can come in varying sizes and shapes, so the point of grammatical correctness is not stamp out creativity or diversity in writing. Rather, grammatical correctness ensures that writing will be enjoyable and clear. One of the most common methods for catching errors is to mouth the words as you read them. Many typos are fixed automatically by our brain, but mouthing the words often circumvents this instinct and helps one read what's actually on the page. Often, grammar errors are caught not by memorization of grammar rules but by the training of one's mind to know whether something *sounds* right or not.

Types of Sentences
There isn't an overabundance of absolutes in grammar, but here is one: every sentence in the English language falls into one of four categories.

- Declarative: a simple statement that ends with a period

  The price of milk per gallon is the same as the price of gasoline.

- Imperative: a command, instruction, or request that ends with a period

  Buy milk when you stop to fill up your car with gas.

- Interrogative: a question that ends with a question mark

  Will you buy the milk?

- Exclamatory: a statement or command that expresses emotions like anger, urgency, or surprise and ends with an exclamation mark

  Buy the milk now!

Declarative sentences are the most common type, probably because they are comprised of the most general content, without any of the bells and whistles that the other three types contain. They are, simply, declarations or statements of any degree of seriousness, importance, or information.

Imperative sentences often seem to be missing a subject. The subject is there, though; it is just not visible or audible because it is *implied*. Look at the imperative example sentence.

  Buy the milk when you fill up your car with gas.

You is the implied subject, the one to whom the command is issued. This is sometimes called *the understood you* because it is understood that *you* is the subject of the sentence.

Interrogative sentences—those that ask questions—are defined as such from the idea of the word *interrogation*, the action of questions being asked of suspects by investigators. Although that is serious business, interrogative sentences apply to all kinds of questions.

To exclaim is at the root of *exclamatory* sentences. These are made with strong emotions behind them. The only technical difference between a declarative or imperative sentence and an exclamatory one is the exclamation mark at the end. The example declarative and imperative sentences can both become an exclamatory one simply by putting an exclamation mark at the end of the sentences.

> The price of milk per gallon is the same as the price of gasoline!
> Buy milk when you stop to fill up your car with gas!

After all, someone might be really excited by the price of gas or milk, or they could be mad at the person that will be buying the milk! However, as stated before, exclamation marks in abundance defeat their own purpose! After a while, they begin to cause fatigue! When used only for their intended purpose, they can have their expected and desired effect.

Lengths

The ideal sentence length—the number of words in a sentence—depends upon the sentence's purpose.

It's okay for a sentence to be brief, and it's fine for a sentence to be lengthy. It's just important to make sure that long sentences do not become run-on sentences or too long to keep up with.

To keep writing interesting, vary sentence lengths, using a mixture of short, medium and long sentences.

Transitions

Transitions are the glue use to make organized thoughts adhere to one another. Transitions are the glue that helps put ideas together seamlessly, within sentences and paragraphs, between them, and (in longer documents) even between sections. Transitions may be single words, sentences, or whole paragraphs (as in the prior example). Transitions help readers to digest and understand what to feel about what has gone on and clue readers in on what is going on, what will be, and how they might react to all these factors. Transitions are like good clues left at a crime scene.

Parallel Structure in a Sentence

Parallel structure, also known as parallelism, refers to using the same grammatical form within a sentence. This is important in lists and for other components of sentences.

> Incorrect: At the recital, the boys and girls were dancing, singing, and played musical instruments.
> Correct: At the recital, the boys and girls were dancing, singing, and playing musical instruments.

Notice that in the second example, *played* is not in the same verb tense as the other verbs nor is it compatible with the helping verb *were*. To test for parallel structure in lists, try reading each item as if it were the only item in the list.

> The boys and girls were dancing.
> The boys and girls were singing.
> The boys and girls were played musical instruments.

Suddenly, the error in the sentence becomes very clear. Here's another example:

> Incorrect: After the accident, I informed the police *that Mrs. Holmes backed* into my car, *that Mrs. Holmes got out* of her car to look at the damage, and *she was driving* off without leaving a note.

> Correct: After the accident, I informed the police *that Mrs. Holmes backed* into my car, *that Mrs. Holmes got out* of her car to look at the damage, and *that Mrs. Holmes drove off* without leaving a note.

Correct: After the accident, I informed the police that Mrs. Holmes *backed* into my car, *got out* of her car to look at the damage, and *drove off* without leaving a note.

Note that there are two ways to fix the nonparallel structure of the first sentence. The key to parallelism is consistent structure.

Examples of Transitional Words and Phrases
Transitions have many emphasis as can be seen below.

- to show emphasis: truly, in fact
- to show examples: for example, namely, specifically
- to show similarities: also, likewise
- to show dissimilarities: on the other hand, even if, in contrast
- to show progression of time: later, previously, subsequently
- to show sequence or order: next, finally
- to show cause and effect: therefore, so
- to show place or position: above, nearby, there
- to provide evidence: furthermore, then
- to summarize: finally, summarizing

Sentence Structures
A *simple sentence* has one independent clause.

I am going to win.

A *compound sentence* has two independent clauses. A conjunction—*for, and, nor, but, or, yet, so*—links them together. Note that each of the independent clauses has a subject and a verb.

I am going to win, but the odds are against me.

A *complex sentence* has one independent clause and one or more dependent clauses.

I am going to win, even though I don't deserve it.

Even though I don't deserve it is a dependent clause. It does not stand on its own. Some conjunctions that link an independent and a dependent clause are *although, because, before, after, that, when, which,* and *while*.

A *compound-complex sentence* has at least three clauses, two of which are independent and at least one that is a dependent clause.

While trying to dance, I tripped over my partner's feet, but I regained my balance quickly.

The dependent clause is *While trying to dance*.

Knowledge of Language

Using Grammar to Enhance Clarity in Writing

<u>Nouns</u>
A noun is a person, place, thing ,or idea. All nouns fit into one of two types, common or proper.

A *common noun* is a word that identifies any of a class of people, places, or things. Examples include numbers, objects, animals, feelings, concepts, qualities, and actions. *A, an,* or *the* usually precedes the common noun. These parts of speech are called *articles*. Here are some examples of sentences using nouns preceded by articles.

> *A* building is under construction.

> *The* girl would like to move to *the* city.

A *proper noun* (also called a *proper name*) is used for the specific name of an individual person, place, or organization. The first letter in a proper noun is capitalized. "My name is *Mary*." "I work for *Walmart*."

Nouns sometimes serve as adjectives (which themselves describe nouns), such as "hockey player" and "state government."

<u>Pronouns</u>
A word used in place of a noun is known as a *pronoun*. Pronouns are words like *I, mine, hers,* and *us*.

Pronouns can be split into different classifications (seen below) which make them easier to learn; however, it's not important to memorize the classifications.

- Personal pronouns: refer to people

- first person: we, I, our, mine

- second person: you, yours

- third person: he, them

- Possessive pronouns: demonstrate ownership (mine, my, his, yours)

- Interrogative pronouns: ask questions (what, which, who, whom, whose)

- Relative pronouns: include the five interrogative pronouns and others that are relative (whoever, whomever, that, when, where)

- Demonstrative pronouns: replace something specific (this, that, those, these)

- Reciprocal pronouns: indicate something was done or given in return (each other, one another)

- Indefinite pronouns: have a nonspecific status (anybody, whoever, someone, everybody, somebody)

Indefinite pronouns such as *anybody, whoever, someone, everybody,* and *somebody* command a singular verb form, but others such as *all, none,* and *some* could require a singular or plural verb form.

209

Antecedents

An *antecedent* is the noun to which a pronoun refers; it needs to be written or spoken before the pronoun is used. For many pronouns, antecedents are imperative for clarity. In particular, a lot of the personal, possessive, and demonstrative pronouns need antecedents. Otherwise, it would be unclear who or what someone is referring to when they use a pronoun like *he* or *this*.

Pronoun reference means that the pronoun should refer clearly to one, clear, unmistakable noun (the antecedent).

Pronoun-antecedent agreement refers to the need for the antecedent and the corresponding pronoun to agree in gender, person, and number. Here are some examples:

The *kidneys* (plural antecedent) are part of the urinary system. *They* (plural pronoun) serve several roles."

The kidneys are part of the *urinary system* (singular antecedent). *It* (singular pronoun) is also known as the renal system.

Pronoun Cases

The subjective pronouns —*I, you, he/she/it, we, they,* and *who*—are the subjects of the sentence.

> Example: *They* have a new house.

The objective pronouns—*me, you* (singular)*, him/her, us, them,* and *whom*—are used when something is being done for or given to someone; they are objects of the action.

> Example: The teacher has an apple for *us*.

The possessive pronouns—*mine, my, your, yours, his, hers, its, their, theirs, our,* and *ours*—are used to denote that something (or someone) belongs to someone (or something).

> Example: It's *their* chocolate cake.

> Even Better Example: It's *my* chocolate cake!

One of the greatest challenges and worst abuses of pronouns concerns *who* and *whom*. Just knowing the following rule can eliminate confusion. *Who* is a subjective-case pronoun used only as a subject or subject complement. *Whom* is only objective-case and, therefore, the object of the verb or preposition.

Hint: When using *who* or *whom*, think of whether someone would say *he* or *him*. If the answer is *he*, use *who*. If the answer is *him*, use *whom*. This trick is easy to remember because *he* and *who* both end in vowels, and *him* and *whom* both end in the letter *M*.

Adjectives

"The *extraordinary* brain is the *main* organ of the central nervous system." The adjective *extraordinary* describes the brain in a way that causes one to realize it is more exceptional than some of other organs while the adjective *main* defines the brain's importance in its system.

An *adjective* is a word or phrase that names an attribute that describes or clarifies a noun or pronoun. This helps the reader visualize and understand the characteristics—size, shape, age, color, origin, etc.—of a person, place, or thing that otherwise might not be known. Adjectives breathe life, color, and depth into the subjects they define. Life would be *drab* and *colorless* without adjectives!

Adjectives often precede the nouns they describe.

> *She drove her <u>new</u> car.*

However, adjectives can also come later in the sentence.

> *Her car is <u>new</u>.*

Adjectives using the prefix *a–* can only be used after a verb.

> Correct: The dog was alive until the car ran up on the curb and hit him.

> Incorrect: The alive dog was hit by a car that ran up on the curb.

Other examples of this rule include *awake, ablaze, ajar, alike,* and *asleep.*

Other adjectives used after verbs concern states of health.

> The girl was finally *well* after a long bout of pneumonia.

> The boy was *fine* after the accident.

An adjective phrase is not a bunch of adjectives strung together, but a group of words that describes a noun or pronoun and, thus, functions as an adjective. *Very ugly* is an adjective phrase; so are *way too fat* and *faster than a speeding bullet.*

Possessives

In grammar, *possessive nouns* show ownership, which was seen in previous examples like *mine, yours,* and *theirs*.

Singular nouns are generally made possessive with an apostrophe and an *s* (*'s*).

> My *uncle's* new car is silver.

> The *dog's* bowl is empty.

> *James's* ties are becoming outdated.

Plural nouns ending in *s* are generally made possessive by just adding an apostrophe (*'*):

> The pistachio nuts' saltiness is added during roasting. (The saltiness of pistachio nuts is added during roasting.)

> The students' achievement tests are difficult. (The achievement tests of the students are difficult.)

If the plural noun does not end in an *s* such as *women,* then it is made possessive by adding an *apostrophe s* (*'s*)—*women's.*

Indefinite possessive pronouns such as *nobody* or *someone* become possessive by adding an *apostrophe s*—*nobody's* or *someone's.*

Verbs

The *verb* is the part of speech that describes an action, state of being, or occurrence.

A *verb* forms the main part of a predicate of a sentence. This means that the verb explains what the noun (which will be discussed shortly) is doing. A simple example is *time flies*. The verb *flies* explains what the action of the noun, *time*, is doing. This example is a *main* verb.

Helping (*auxiliary*) verbs are words like *have, do, be, can, may, should, must,* and *will.* "I *should* go to the store." Helping verbs assist main verbs in expressing tense, ability, possibility, permission, or obligation.

Particles are minor function words like *not, in, out, up,* or *down* that become part of the verb itself. "I might *not.*"

Participles are words formed from verbs that are often used to modify a noun, noun phrase, verb, or verb phrase.

> The *running* teenager collided with the cyclist.

Participles can also create compound verb forms.

> He is *speaking*.

Verbs have five basic forms: the *base* form, the *-s* form, the *-ing* form, the *past* form, and the *past participle* form.

The *past* forms are either *regular* (*love/loved; hate/hated*) or *irregular* because they don't end by adding the common past tense suffix "-ed" (*go/went; fall/fell; set/set*).

Adverbs
Adverbs have more functions than adjectives because they modify or qualify verbs, adjectives, or other adverbs as well as word groups that express a relation of place, time, circumstance, or cause. Therefore, adverbs answer any of the following questions: *How, when, where, why, in what way, how often, how much, in what condition, and/or to what degree. How good looking is he? He is very handsome.*

Here are some examples of adverbs for different situations:

- how: quickly
- when: daily
- where: there
- in what way: easily
- how often: often
- how much: much
- in what condition: badly
- what degree: hardly

As one can see, for some reason, many adverbs end in *-ly.*

Adverbs do things like emphasize (*really, simply,* and *so*), amplify (*heartily, completely,* and *positively*), and tone down (*almost, somewhat,* and *mildly*).

Adverbs also come in phrases.

> The dog ran as though his life depended on it.

Prepositions

Prepositions are connecting words and, while there are only about 150 of them, they are used more often than any other individual groups of words. They describe relationships between other words. They are placed before a noun or pronoun, forming a phrase that modifies another word in the sentence. *Prepositional phrases* begin with a preposition and end with a noun or pronoun, the *object of the preposition. A pristine lake is <u>near the store</u> and <u>behind the bank.</u>*

Some commonly used prepositions are *about, after, anti, around, as, at, behind, beside, by, for, from, in, into, of, off, on, to,* and *with.*

Complex prepositions, which also come before a noun or pronoun, consist of two or three words such as *according to, in regards to,* and *because of.*

Interjections

Interjections are words used to express emotion. Examples include *wow, ouch,* and *hooray.* Interjections are often separate from sentences; in those cases, the interjection is directly followed by an exclamation point. In other cases the interjection is included in a sentence and followed by a comma. The punctuation plays a big role in the intensity of the emotion that the interjection is expressing. Using a comma or semicolon indicates less excitement than using an exclamation mark

Conjunctions

Conjunctions are vital words that connect words, phrases, thoughts, and ideas. Conjunctions show relationships between components. There are two types:

Coordinating conjunctions are the primary class of conjunctions placed between words, phrases, clauses, and sentences that are of equal grammatical rank; the coordinating conjunctions are *or, and, nor, but, or, yes,* and *so.* A useful memorization trick is to remember that the first letter of these conjunctions collectively spell the word *fanboys.*

I need to go shopping, *but* I must be careful to leave enough money in the bank.

She wore a black, red, *and* white shirt.

Subordinating conjunctions are the secondary class of conjunctions. They connect two unequal parts, one *main* (or *independent*) and the other *subordinate* (or *dependent*). I must go to the store *even though* I do not have enough money in the bank.

Because I read the review, I do not want to go to the movie.

Notice that the presence of subordinating conjunctions makes clauses dependent. *I read the movie* is an independent clause, but *because* makes the clause dependent. Thus, it needs an independent clause to complete the sentence.

Subject-Verb Agreement

The subject of a sentence and its verb must agree. The cornerstone rule of subject-verb agreement is that subject and verb must agree in number. Whether the subject is singular or plural, the verb must follow suit.

Incorrect: The houses is new.

Correct: The houses are new.

Also Correct: The house is new.

In other words, a singular subject requires a singular verb; a plural subject requires a plural verb.

The words or phrases that come between the subject and verb do not alter this rule.

>Incorrect: The houses built of brick is new.

>Correct: The houses built of brick are new.

>Incorrect: The houses with the sturdy porches is new.

>Correct: The houses with the sturdy porches are new.

The subject will always follow the verb when a sentence begins with *here* or *there*. Identify these with care.

>Incorrect: Here *is* the *houses* with sturdy porches.

>Correct: Here *are* the *houses* with sturdy porches.

The subject in the sentences above is not *here*, it is *houses*. Remember, *here* and *there* are never subjects. Be careful that contractions such as *here's* or *there're* do not cause confusion!

Two subjects joined by *and* require a plural verb form, except when the two combine to make one thing:

>Incorrect: Garrett and Jonathan is over there.

>Correct: Garrett and Jonathan are over there.

>Incorrect: Spaghetti and meatballs are a delicious meal!

>Correct: Spaghetti and meatballs is a delicious meal!

In the example above, *spaghetti and meatballs* is a compound noun. However, *Garrett and Jonathan* is not a compound noun.

Two singular subjects joined by *or, either/or,* or *neither/nor* call for a singular verb form.

>Incorrect: Butter or syrup are acceptable.

>Correct: Butter or syrup is acceptable.

Plural subjects joined by *or, either/or,* or *neither/nor* are, indeed, plural.

The chairs or the boxes are being moved next.

If one subject is singular and the other is plural, the verb should agree with the closest noun.

>Correct: The chair or the boxes are being moved next.

>Correct: The chairs or the box is being moved next.

Some plurals of money, distance, and time call for a singular verb.

>Incorrect: Three dollars *are* enough to buy that.

>Correct: Three dollars *is* enough to buy that.

For words declaring degrees of quantity such as *many of, some of,* or *most of,* let the noun that follows *of* be the guide:.

Incorrect: Many of the books is in the shelf.

Correct: Many of the books are in the shelf.

Incorrect: Most of the pie *are* on the table.

Correct: Most of the pie *is* on the table.

For indefinite pronouns like anybody or everybody, use singular verbs.

Everybody *is* going to the store.

However, the pronouns *few, many, several, all, some,* and *both* have their own rules and use plural forms.

Some *are* ready.

Some nouns like *crowd* and *congress* are called *collective nouns* and they require a singular verb form.

Congress *is* in session.

The news *is* over.

Books and movie titles, though, including plural nouns such as *Great Expectations*, also require a singular verb. Remember that only the subject affects the verb. While writing tricky subject-verb arrangements, say them aloud. Listen to them. Once the rules have been learned, one's ear will become sensitive to them, making it easier to pick out what's right and what's wrong.

Distinguishing Between Formal and Informal Language

It can be helpful to distinguish whether a writer or speaker is using formal or informal language because it can give the reader or listener clues to whether the text is informative, non-fiction, argumentative, or the intended tone or audience. Formal and informal language in written or verbal communication serve different purposes and are often intended for different audiences. Consequently, their tone, word choices, and grammatical structures vary. These differences can be used to identify which form of language is used in a given piece and to determine which type of language should be used for a certain context. Understanding the differences between formal and informal language will also allow a writer or speaker to implement the most appropriate and effective style for a given situation.

Formal language is less personal and more informative and pragmatic than informal language. It is more "buttoned-up" and business-like, adhering to proper grammatical rules. It is used in professional or academic contexts, to convey respect or authority. For example, one would use formal language to write an informative or argumentative essay for school and to address a superior or esteemed professional like a potential employer, a professor, or a manager. Formal language avoids contractions, slang, colloquialisms, and first person pronouns. *Slang* refers to non-standard expressions that are not used in elevated speech and writing. Slang creates linguistic in-groups and out-groups of people, those who can understand the slang terms and those who can't. Slang is often tied to a specific time period. For example, "groovy" and "far out" are connected to the 1970s, and "as if!" and "4-1-1-" are connected to the 1990s. *Colloquial* language is language that is used conversationally or familiarly—e.g., "What's up?"—in contrast to formal, professional, or academic language—"How are you this evening?" Formal language uses sentences that are usually more complex and often in passive voice.

Punctuation can differ as well. For example, *exclamation point (!)* are used to show strong emotion or can be used as an *interjection* but should be used sparingly in formal writing situations.

Informal language is often used when communicating with family members, friends, peers, and those known more personally. It is more casual, spontaneous, and forgiving in its conformity to grammatical rules and conventions. Informal language is used for personal emails, some light fiction stories, and some correspondence between coworkers or other familial relationships. The tone is more relaxed and slang, contractions, clichés, and the first and second person may be used in writing. The imperative voice may be used as well.

As a review, the perspectives from which something may be written or conveyed are detailed below:

- *First-person point of view*: The story is told from the writer's perspective. In fiction, this would mean that the main character is also the narrator. First-person point of view is easily recognized by the use of personal pronouns such as *I, me, we, us, our, my,* and *myself*.

- *Second-person point of view*: This point of view isn't commonly used in fiction or non-fiction writing because it directly addresses the reader using the pronouns you, your, and yourself. Second-person perspective is more appropriate in direct communication, such as business letters or emails.

- *Third-person point of view*: In a more formal essay, this would be an appropriate perspective because the focus should be on the subject matter, not the writer or the reader. Third-person point of view is recognized by the use of the pronouns *he, she, they,* and *it*. In fiction writing, third person point of view has a few variations.

  o *Third-person limited* point of view refers to a story told by a narrator who has access to the thoughts and feelings of just one character.

  o In *third-person omniscient* point of view, the narrator has access to the thoughts and feelings of all the characters.

  o In *third-person objective* point of view, the narrator is like a fly on the wall and can see and hear what the characters do and say, but does not have access to their thoughts and feelings.

Applying Basic Knowledge of the Elements of the Writing Process

Practice Makes Prepared Writers
Like any other useful skill, writing only improves with practice. While writing may come more easily to some than others, it is still a skill to be honed and improved. Regardless of a person's natural abilities, there is always room for growth in writing. Practicing the basic skills of writing can aid in preparations for the TEAS.

One way to build vocabulary and enhance exposure to the written word is through reading. This can be through reading books, but reading of any materials such as newspapers, magazines, and even social media count towards practice with the written word. This also helps to enhance critical reading and thinking skills, through analysis of the ideas and concepts read. Think of each new reading experience as a chance to sharpen these skills.

Planning
Brainstorming
One of the most important steps in writing an essay is prewriting. Before drafting an essay, it's helpful to think about the topic for a moment or two, in order to gain a more solid understanding of what the task is. Then, spending about five minutes jotting down the immediate ideas that could work for the essay is recommended.

Brainstorming is a way to get some words on the page and offer a reference for ideas when drafting. Scratch paper is provided for writers to use any prewriting techniques such as webbing, free writing, or listing. The goal is to get ideas out of the mind and onto the page.

Once the ideas are on the page, it's time to turn them into a solid plan for the essay. The best ideas from the brainstorming results can then be developed into a more formal outline.

Outlining
An *outline* is a system used to organize writing. When reading texts, outlining is important because it helps readers organize important information in a logical pattern using Roman numerals. Usually, outlines start out with the main idea(s) and then branch out into subgroups or subsidiary thoughts or subjects. The outline should be methodical, with at least two main points follow each by at least two subpoints. Not only do outlines provide a visual tool for readers to reflect on how events, characters, settings, or other key parts of the text or passage relate to one another, but they can also lead readers to a stronger conclusion. The sample below demonstrates what a general outline looks like.

I.   Main Topic 1
   a.   Subtopic 1
   b.   Subtopic 2
      1.   Detail 1
      2.   Detail 2
II. Main Topic 2
   a.   Subtopic 1
   b.   Subtopic 2
      1.   Detail 1
      2.   Detail 2

Free Writing
Like brainstorming, free writing is another prewriting activity to help the writer generate ideas. This method involves setting a timer for 2 or 3 minutes and writing down all ideas that come to mind about the topic using complete sentences. Once time is up, review the sentences to see what observations have been made and how these ideas might translate into a more coherent direction for the topic. Even if sentences lack sense as a whole, this is an excellent way to get ideas onto the page in the very beginning stages of writing. Using complete sentences can make this a bit more challenging than brainstorming, but overall it is a worthwhile exercise, as it may force the writer to come up with more complete thoughts about the topic.

Writing
Now it comes time to actually write your essay. Follow the outline you developed in the brainstorming process and try to incorporate the sentences you wrote in the free writing exercise.

Remember that your work here does not have to be perfect. This process is often referred to as *drafting* because you're just creating a rough draft of your work.

Don't get bogged down on the small details. For instance, if you're not sure whether or not a word should be capitalized, mark it somehow and look up the capitalization rule while in the revision process. The same goes for referencing sources. That should not be focused on until after the writing process.

<u>Referencing Sources</u>

Anytime you quote or paraphrase another piece of writing you will need to include a citation. A citation is a short description of the work that your quote or information came from. The manual of style your teacher wants you to follow will dictate exactly how to format that citation. For example, this is how you would cite a book according to the APA manual of style:

- *Format*: Last name, First initial, Middle initial. (Year Published) *Book Title*. City, State: Publisher.
- *Example*: Sampson, M. R. (1989). *Diaries from an alien invasion*. Springfield, IL: Campbell Press.

<u>Revising</u>

Revising and proofreading offers an opportunity for writers to polish things up. Putting one's self in the reader's shoes and focusing on what the essay actually says helps writers identify problems—it's a movement from the mindset of writer to the mindset of editor. The goal is to have a clean, clear copy of the essay. The following areas should be considered when proofreading:

- Sentence fragments
- Awkward sentence structure
- Run-on sentences
- Incorrect word choice
- Grammatical agreement errors
- Spelling errors
- Punctuation errors
- Capitalization errors

<u>Recursive Writing Process</u>

While the writing process may have specific steps, the good news is that the process is recursive, meaning the steps need not be completed in a particular order. Many writers find that they complete steps at the same time such as drafting and revising, where the writing and rearranging of ideas occur simultaneously or in very close order. Similarly, a writer may find that a particular section of a draft needs more development, and will go back to the prewriting stage to generate new ideas. The steps can be repeated at any time, and the more these steps of the recursive writing process are employed, the better the final product will be.

Developing a Well-Organized Paragraph

<u>Forming Paragraphs</u>

A good *paragraph* should have the following characteristics:

- be logical with organized sentences
- have a *unified* purpose within itself
- use sentences as *building blocks*
- be a *distinct section* of a piece of writing
- present a *single theme* introduced by a *topic sentence*
- maintain a *consistent flow* through subsequent, relevant, well-placed sentences
- *tell a story* of its own or have its own purpose, yet connect with what is written before and after
- enlighten, entertain, and/or inform

Though certainly not set in stone, the length should be a consideration for the reader's sake, not merely for the sake of the topic. When paragraphs are especially short, the reader might experience an irregular, uneven effect; when they're much longer than 250 words, the reader's attention span, and probably their retention, is challenged. While a paragraph can technically be a sentence long, a good rule of thumb is for paragraphs to be at least three sentences long and no more than ten sentence long. An optimal word length is 100 to 250 words.

Coherent Paragraphs

Coherence is simply defined as the quality of being logical and consistent. In order to have coherent paragraphs, therefore, authors must be logical and consistent in their writing, whatever the document might be. Two words are helpful to understanding coherence: flow and relationship. Earlier, transitions were referred to as being the "glue" to put organized thoughts together. Now, let's look at the topic sentence from which flow and relationship originate.

The topic sentence, usually the first in a paragraph, holds the essential features that will be brought forth in the paragraph. Not only is it important because of what it is and contains but also because it is here that authors either grab or lose readers. It also may be the only piece that a reader encounters from that writer, so it is a good idea to summarize and represent ideas accurately.

The coherent paragraph has a logical order. It utilizes transitional words and phrases, parallel sentence structure, clear pronoun references, and reasonable repetition of key words and phrases. Use common sense for repetition. Consider synonyms for variety. Be consistent in verb tense whenever possible.

When writers have accomplished their paragraph's purpose, they prepare it to receive the next. While writing, read the paragraph over, edit, examine, evaluate, and make changes accordingly. Possibly, a paragraph has gone on too long. If that occurs, it needs to be broken up into other paragraphs, or the length should be reduced. If a paragraph didn't fully accomplish its purpose, consider it a chance for revisions. One might simply say, "Ah, that is good."

Main Point of a Paragraph

What is the main point of a paragraph? It is *the* point all of the other important and lesser important points should lead up to, and it should be summed up in the topic sentence.

Sometimes there is a fine line of difference to distinguish between a paragraph's topic sentence and its main point because of their relationship. In fact, they actually might be one and the same. Often, though, they are two separate but closely related aspects of the same paragraph.

Depending upon writers' purposes, they might not fully reveal the topic sentence or the paragraph's main point until the paragraph's conclusion.

Sometimes, while developing paragraphs, authors deviate from the main point, which means they have to delete and rework their materials to stay on point.

Examining Paragraphs

Throughout this text, composing and combining sentences, using basic grammar skills, employing rules and guidelines, identifying differing points of view, using appropriate context, constructing accurate word usage, and discerning correct punctuation have all been discussed. Whew! The types of sentences, patterns, transitions, and overall structure have been covered as well.

While authors write, thoughts coalesce to form words on "paper" (aka a computer screen). Authors strategically place those thoughts in sentences to give them "voice" in an orderly manner, and then they manipulate them into cohesive sentences for cohesion to express ideas. Like a hunk of modeling clay (thanks to computers, people are no longer bound to erasers and whiteout), sentences can be worked and reworked until they cooperate and say what was originally intended.

Before calling a paragraph complete, identify its main point, making sure that related sentences stay on point. Pose questions such as, "Did I sufficiently develop the main point by the other points pointing to it? Did I say it succinctly enough? Did I give it time to develop? *Is* it developed?"

Let's examine the following two paragraphs, each an example of a movie review. Read them and form a critique.

Example 1: *Eddie the Eagle* is a movie about a struggling athlete. Eddie was crippled at birth. He had a lot of therapy and he had a dream. Eddie trained himself for the Olympics. He went far away to learn how to ski jump. It was hard for him, but he persevered. He got a coach and kept trying. He qualified for the Olympics. He was the only one from Britain who could jump. When he succeeded, they named him, "Eddie the Eagle."

Example 2: The last movie I saw in the theater was *Eddie the Eagle,* a story of extraordinary perseverance inspired by real life events. Eddie was born in England with a birth defect that he slowly but surely overcame, but not without trial and error (not the least of which was his father's perpetual *dis*couragement). In fact, the old man did everything to get him to give up, but Eddie was dogged beyond anyone in the neighborhood; in fact, maybe beyond anyone in the whole town or even the whole world! Eddie, simply, did not know to quit. As he grew up, so did his dream; a strange one, indeed, for someone so unaccomplished: to compete in the Winter Olympics as a ski jumper (which he knew absolutely nothing about). Eddie didn't just keep on dreaming about it. He actually went to Germany and *worked* at it, facing unbelievable odds, defeats, and put-downs by Dad and the other Men in Charge, aka the Olympic decision-makers. Did that stop him? No way! Eddie got a coach and persevered. Then, when he failed, he persevered some more, again and again. You should be able to open up a dictionary, look at the word "persevere," and see a picture of Eddie the Eagle because, when everybody told him he couldn't, he did. The result? He is forever dubbed, "Eddie the Eagle."

Both reviews tell something about the movie *Eddie the Eagle*. Does one motivate the reader to want to see the movie more than the other? Does one just provide a few facts while the other paints a virtual picture of the movie? Does one give a carrot and the other a rib eye steak, mashed potatoes, and chocolate silk pie?

Paragraphs sometimes only give facts. Sometimes that's appropriate and all that is needed. Sometimes, though, writers want to use the blank documents on their computer screens to paint a picture. Writers must "see" the painting come to life. To do so, pick a familiar topic, write a simple sentence, and add to it. Pretend, for instance, there's a lovely view. What does one see? Is it a lake? Try again – picture it as though it were the sea! Visualize a big ship sailing out there. Is it sailing away or approaching ? Who is on it? Is it dangerous? Is it night and are there crazy pirates on board? Uh-oh! Did one just jump ship and start swimming toward shore?

Vocabulary Acquisition

Using Context Clues to Determine the Meaning of Words or Phrases

Context clues help readers understand unfamiliar words, and thankfully, there are many types.

Synonyms are words or phrases that have nearly, if not exactly, the same meaning as other words or phrases

> *Large* boxes are needed to pack *big* items.

Antonyms are words or phrases that have opposite definitions. Antonyms, like synonyms, can serve as context clues, although more cryptically.

> *Large* boxes are not needed to pack *small* items.

Definitions are sometimes included within a sentence to define uncommon words.

> They practiced the *rumba*, a *type of dance*, for hours on end.

Explanations provide context through elaboration.

> Large boxes holding items weighing over 60 pounds were stacked in the corner.

Here's an example of *contrast*:

> These *minute* creatures were much different than the *huge* mammals that the zoologist was accustomed to dealing with.

Determining the Meaning of Words by Analyzing Word Parts

By analyzing and understanding Latin, Greek, and Anglo-Saxon word roots, prefixes, and suffixes one can better understand word meanings. Of course, people can always look words up if a dictionary or thesaurus if available, but meaning can often be gleaned on the spot if the writer learns to dissect and examine words.

A word can consist of the following:

- root
- root + suffix
- prefix + root
- prefix + root + suffix

For example, if someone was unfamiliar with the word *submarine* they could break the word into its parts.

> prefix + root
> sub + marine

It can be determined that *sub* means *below* as in *subway* and *subpar*. Additionally, one can determine that *marine* refers to *the sea* as in *marine life*. Thus, it can be figured that *submarine* refers to something below the water.

Roots

Roots are the basic components of words. Many roots can stand alone as individual words, but others must be combined with a prefix or suffix to be a word. For example, *calc* is a root but it needs a suffix to be an actual word (*calcium*).

Prefixes

A *prefix* is a word, letter, or number that is placed before another. It adjusts or qualifies the root word's meaning. When written alone, prefixes are followed by a dash to indicate that the root word follows. Some of the most common prefixes are the following:

Prefix	Meaning	Example
dis-	not or opposite of	disabled
in-, im-, il-, ir-	not	illiterate
re-	again	return
un-	not	unpredictable
anti-	against	antibacterial
fore-	before	forefront
mis-	wrongly	misunderstand
non-	not	nonsense
over-	more than normal	overabundance
pre-	before	preheat
super-	above	superman

Suffixes

A suffix is a letter or group of letters added at the end of a word to form another word. The word created from the root and suffix is either a different tense of the same root (*help* + *ed* = *helped*) or a new word (*help* + *ful* = *helpful*). When written alone, suffixes are preceded by a dash to indicate that the root word comes before.

Some of the most common suffixes are the following:

Suffix	Meaning	Example
ed	makes a verb past tense	wash*ed*
ing	makes a verb a present participle verb	wash*ing*
ly	to make characteristic of	love*ly*
s/es	to make more than one	chair*s*, box*es*
able	can be done	deplor*able*
al	having characteristics of	comic*al*
est	comparative	great*est*
ful	full of	wonder*ful*
ism	belief in	commun*ism*
less	without	faith*less*
ment	action or process	accomplish*ment*
ness	state of	happi*ness*
ize, ise	to render, to make	steril*ize*, advert*ise*
cede/ceed/sede	go	con*cede*, pro*ceed*, super*sede*

Here are some helpful tips:

- When adding a suffix that starts with a vowel (for example, -ed) to a one-syllable root whose vowel has a short sound and ends in a consonant (for example, *stun*), double the final consonant of the root (*n*).

    stun + ed = stun*n*ed

    Exception: If the past tense verb ends in *x* such as *box*, do not double the *x*.

    box + ed = boxed

- If adding a suffix that starts with a vowel (-er) to a multi-syllable word ending in a consonant (*begin*), double the consonant (*n*).

    begin + er = begin*n*er

- If a short vowel is followed by two or more consonants in a word such as *i+t+c+h = itch,* do <u>not</u> double the last consonant.

    itch + ed = itched

- If adding a suffix that starts with a vowel (-*ing*) to a word ending in *e* (for example, *name*), that word's final *e* is generally (but not always) dropped.

    name + ing = naming
    exception: manage + able = manag*e*able

- If adding a suffix that starts with a consonant (-*ness*) to a word ending in *e* (*complete*), the *e* generally (but not always) remains.

    complete + ness = completeness
    exception: judge + ment = judgment

There is great diversity on handling words that end in *y*. For words ending in a vowel + *y*, nothing changes in the original word.

    play + ed = played

For words ending in a consonant + *y*, change the *y* to *i* when adding any suffix except for –*ing*.

    marry + ed = married
    marry + ing = marrying

Practice Questions

1. Which of the following sentences has an error in capitalization?
    a. The East Coast has experienced very unpredictable weather this year.
    b. My Uncle owns a home in Florida, where he lives in the winter.
    c. I am taking English Composition II on campus this fall.
    d. There are several nice beaches we can visit on our trip to the Jersey Shore this summer.

2. Julia Robinson, an avid photographer in her spare time, was able to capture stunning shots of the local wildlife on her last business trip to Australia.
Which of the following is an adjective in the preceding sentence?
    a. Time
    b. Capture
    c. Avid
    d. Photographer

3. Which of the following sentences uses correct punctuation?
    a. Carole is not currently working; her focus is on her children at the moment.
    b. Carole is not currently working and her focus is on her children at the moment.
    c. Carole is not currently working, her focus is on her children at the moment.
    d. Carole is not currently working her focus is on her children at the moment.

4. Which of these examples is a compound sentence?
    a. Alex and Shane spent the morning coloring and later took a walk down to the park.
    b. After coloring all morning, Alex and Shane spent the afternoon at the park.
    c. Alex and Shane spent the morning coloring, and then they took a walk down to the park.
    d. After coloring all morning and spending part of the day at the park, Alex and Shane took a nap.

5. Which of these examples shows incorrect use of subject-verb agreement?
    a. Neither of the cars are parked on the street.
    b. Both of my kids are going to camp this summer.
    c. Any of your friends are welcome to join us on the trip in November.
    d. Each of the clothing options is appropriate for the job interview.

6. When it gets warm in the spring, _____ and _____ like to go fishing at Cobbs Creek.
Which of the following word pairs should be used in the blanks above?
    a. me, him
    b. he, I
    c. him, I
    d. he, me

7. Which example shows correct comma usage for dates?
    a. The due date for the final paper in the course is Monday, May 16, 2016.
    b. The due date for the final paper in the course is Monday, May 16 2016.
    c. The due date for the final project in the course is Monday, May, 16, 2016.
    d. The due date for the final project in the course is Monday May 16, 2016.

8. Which of the following uses correct spelling?

a. Leslie knew that training for the Philadelphia Marathon would take dicsipline and perserverance, but she was up to the challenge.

b. Leslie knew that training for the Philadelphia Marathon would take discipline and perseverence, but she was up to the challenge.

c. Leslie knew that training for the Philadelphia Marathon would take disiplin and perservearance, but she was up to the challenge.

d. Leslie knew that training for the Philadelphia Marathon would take discipline and perseverance, but she was up to the challenge.

9. At last night's company function, in honor of Mr. Robertson's retirement, several employees spoke kindly about his career achievements.

In the preceding sentence, what part of speech is the word *function*?

a. Adjective

b. Adverb

c. Verb

d. Noun

10. Which of the examples uses the correct plural form?

a. Tomatos

b. Analysis

c. Cacti

d. Criterion

11. Which of the following examples uses correct punctuation?

a. The moderator asked the candidates, "Is each of you prepared to discuss your position on global warming?".

b. The moderator asked the candidates, "Is each of you prepared to discuss your position on global warming?"

c. The moderator asked the candidates, 'Is each of you prepared to discuss your position on global warming?'

d. The moderator asked the candidates, "Is each of you prepared to discuss your position on global warming"?

12. Based on the words *transfer, transact, translation, transport*, what is the meaning of the prefix *trans*?

a. Separation

b. All, everywhere

c. Forward

d. Across, beyond, over

13. In which of the following sentences does the word *part* function as an adjective?

a. The part Brian was asked to play required many hours of research.

b. She parts ways with the woodsman at the end of the book.

c. The entire team played a part in the success of the project.

d. Ronaldo is part Irish on his mother's side of the family.

14. All of Shannon's family and friends helped her to celebrate her 50th birthday at Café Sorrento.
Which of the following is the complete subject of the preceding sentence?
    a. Family and friends
    b. All
    c. All of Shannon's family and friends
    d. Shannon's family and friends

15. Which of the following sentences uses second person point of view?
    a. I don't want to make plans for the weekend before I see my work schedule.
    b. She had to miss the last three yoga classes due to illness.
    c. Pluto is no longer considered a planet because it is not gravitationally dominant.
    d. Be sure to turn off all of the lights before locking up for the night.

16. As the tour group approached the bottom of Chichen Itza, the prodigious Mayan pyramid, they became nervous about climbing its distant peak.

Based on the context of the sentence, which of the following words shows the correct meaning of the word *prodigious*?
    a. Very large
    b. Famous
    c. Very old
    d. Fancy

17. Which of the following sentences correctly uses a hyphen?
    a. Last-year, many of the players felt unsure of the coach's methods.
    b. Some of the furniture she selected seemed a bit over - the - top for the space.
    c. Henry is a beagle-mix and is ready for adoption this weekend.
    d. Geena works to maintain a good relationship with her ex-husband to the benefit of their children.

18. Which of the following examples correctly uses quotation marks?
    a. "A Wrinkle in Time" was one of my favorite novels as a child.
    b. Though he is famous for his roles in films like "The Great Gatsby" and "Titanic," Leonardo DiCaprio has never won an Oscar.
    c. Sylvia Plath's poem, "Daddy" will be the subject of this week's group discussion.
    d. "The New York Times" reported that many fans are disappointed in some of the trades made by the Yankees this off-season.

19. Which of the following sentences shows correct word usage?
    a. It's often been said that work is better then rest.
    b. Its often been said that work is better then rest.
    c. It's often been said that work is better than rest.
    d. Its often been said that work is better than rest.

20. Glorify, fortify, gentrify, acidify

Based on the preceding words, what is the correct meaning of the suffix *–fy*?
    a. Marked by, given to
    b. Doer, believer
    c. Make, cause, cause to have
    d. Process, state, rank

21. Which of the following uses correct spelling?
    a. Jed was disatisfied with the acommodations at his hotel, so he requested another room.
    b. Jed was dissatisfied with the accommodations at his hotel, so he requested another room.
    c. Jed was dissatisfied with the accomodations at his hotel, so he requested another room.
    d. Jed was disatisfied with the accommodations at his hotel, so he requested another room.

22. Which of the following is an imperative sentence?
    a. Pennsylvania's state flag includes two draft horses and an eagle.
    b. Go down to the basement and check the hot water heater for signs of a leak.
    c. You must be so excited to have a new baby on the way!
    d. How many countries speak Spanish?

23. After a long day at work, Tracy had dinner with her family, and then took a walk to the park.
What are the transitional words in the preceding sentence?
    a. After, then
    b. At, with, to
    c. Had, took
    d. A, the

24. Which of the following examples is a compound sentence?
    a. Shawn and Jerome played soccer in the backyard for two hours.
    b. Marissa last saw Elena and talked to her this morning.
    c. The baby was sick, so I decided to stay home from work.
    d. Denise, Kurt, and Eric went for a run after dinner.

25. Robert needed to find at least four sources for his final project, so he searched several library databases for reliable academic research.
Which words function as nouns in the preceding sentence?
    a. Robert, sources, project, databases, research
    b. Robert, sources, final, project, databases, academic, research
    c. Robert, sources, project, he, library, databases, research
    d. Sources, project, databases, research

26. Which of the following sentences uses correct subject-verb agreement?
    a. There is two constellations that can be seen from the back of the house.
    b. At least four of the sheep needs to be sheared before the end of summer.
    c. Lots of people were auditioning for the singing competition on Saturday.
    d. Everyone in the group have completed the assignment on time.

27. Philadelphia is home to some excellent walking tours where visitors can learn more about the culture and rich history of the city of brotherly love.
What are the adjectives in the preceding sentence?
    a. Philadelphia, tours, visitors, culture, history, city, love
    b. Excellent, walking, rich, brotherly
    c. Is, can, learn
    d. To, about, of

28. The realtor showed _____ and _____ a house on Wednesday afternoon.
Which of the following pronoun pairs should be used in the blanks above?
    a. She, I
    b. She, me
    c. Me, her
    d. Her, me

29. Which of the following examples uses correct punctuation?
    a. Recommended supplies for the hunting trip include the following: rain gear, large backpack, hiking boots, flashlight, and non-perishable foods.
    b. I left the store, because I forgot my wallet.
    c. As soon as the team checked into the hotel; they met in the lobby for a group photo.
    d. None of the furniture came in on time: so they weren't able to move in to the new apartment.

30. Which of the following sentences shows correct word usage?
    a. Your going to have to put you're jacket over their.
    b. You're going to have to put your jacket over there.
    c. Your going to have to put you're jacket over they're.
    d. You're going to have to put you're jacket over their.

31. A student wants to rewrite the following sentence:
      Entrepreneurs use their ideas to make money.

He wants to use the word *money* as a verb, but he isn't sure which word ending to use. What is the appropriate suffix to add to *money* to complete the following sentence?

                        Entrepreneurs _____ *their ideas.*

    a. –ize
    b. –ical
    c. –en
    d. –ful

32. A teacher notices that, when students are talking to each other between classes, they are using their own unique vocabulary words and expressions to talk about their daily lives. When the teacher hears these non-standard words that are specific to one age or cultural group, what type of language is she listening to?
    a. Slang
    b. Jargon
    c. Dialect
    d. Vernacular

33. A teacher wants to counsel a student about using the word *ain't* in a research paper for a high school English class. What advice should the teacher give?
    a. *Ain't* is not in the dictionary, so it isn't a word.
    b. Because the student isn't in college yet, *ain't* is an appropriate expression for a high school writer.
    c. *Ain't* is incorrect English and should not be part of a serious student's vocabulary because it sounds uneducated.
    d. *Ain't* is a colloquial expression, and while it may be appropriate in a conversational setting, it is not standard in academic writing.

228

Use the passage below for questions 2 through 5:

<u>Caribbean Island Destinations</u>

Do you want to vacation at a Caribbean island destination? Who wouldn't want a tropical vacation? Visit one of the many Caribbean islands where visitors can swim in crystal blue waters, swim with dolphins, or enjoy family-friendly or adult-only resorts and activities. Every island offers a unique and picturesque vacation destination. Choose from these islands: Aruba, St. Lucia, Barbados, Anguilla, St. John, and so many more. A Caribbean island destination will be the best and most refreshing vacation ever . . . no regrets!

34. What is the topic of the passage?
    a. Caribbean island destinations
    b. Tropical vacation
    c. Resorts
    d. Activities

35. What is/are the supporting detail(s) of this passage?
    a. Cruising to the Caribbean
    b. Local events
    c. Family or adult-only resorts and activities
    d. All of the above

36. Taylor is working on an essay and is trying to put topics determined during brainstorming into a good order for her paper. What element of the writing process is she working on?
    a. Organizing
    b. Drafting
    c. Revising
    d. Outlining

Answer Explanations

1. B: In choice B the word *Uncle* should not be capitalized, because it is not functioning as a proper noun. If the word named a specific uncle, such as *Uncle Jerry*, then it would be considered a proper noun and should be capitalized. Choice *A* correctly capitalizes the proper noun *East Coast*, and does not capitalize *winter*, which functions as a common noun in the sentence. Choice *C* correctly capitalizes the name of a specific college course, which is considered a proper noun. Choice *D* correctly capitalizes the proper noun *Jersey Shore*.

2. C: In choice C, *avid* is functioning as an adjective that modifies the word photographer. *Avid* describes the photographer Julia Robinson's style. The words *time* and *photographer* are functioning as nouns, and the word *capture* is functioning as a verb in the sentence. Other words functioning as adjectives in the sentence include, *local*, *business*, and *spare*, as they all describe the nouns they precede.

3. A: Choice *A* is correctly punctuated because it uses a semicolon to join two independent clauses that are related in meaning. Each of these clauses could function as an independent sentence. Choice *B* is incorrect because the conjunction is not preceded by a comma. A comma and conjunction should be used together to join independent clauses. Choice *C* is incorrect because a comma should only be used to join independent sentences when it also includes a coordinating conjunction such as *and* or *so*. Choice *D* does not use punctuation to join the independent clauses, so it is considered a fused (same as a run-on) sentence.

4. C: Choice *C* is a compound sentence because it joins two independent clauses with a comma and the coordinating conjunction *and*. The sentences in Choices B and D include one independent clause and one dependent clause, so they are complex sentences, not compound sentences. The sentence in Choice A has both a compound subject, *Alex and Shane*, and a compound verb, *spent and took*, but the entire sentence itself is one independent clause.

5. A: Choice *A* uses incorrect subject-verb agreement because the indefinite pronoun *neither* is singular and must use the singular verb form *is*. The pronoun *both* is plural and uses the plural verb form of *are*. The pronoun *any* can be either singular or plural. In this example, it is used as a plural, so the plural verb form *are* is used. The pronoun *each* is singular and uses the singular verb form *is*.

6. B: Choice *B* is correct because the pronouns *he* and *I* are in the subjective case. *He* and *I* are the subjects of the verb *like* in the independent clause of the sentence. Choice A, C, and D are incorrect because they all contain at least one objective pronoun (*me* and *him*). Objective pronouns should not be used as the subject of the sentence, but rather, they should come as an object of a verb. To test for correct pronoun usage, try reading the pronouns as if it were the only pronoun in the sentence. For example, *he* and *me* may appear to be the correct answer choices, but try reading them as the only pronoun.

> He like[s] to go fishing…

> Me like to go fishing…

> When looked at that way, *me* is an obviously incorrect choice.

7. A: It is necessary to put a comma between the date and the year. It is also required to put a comma between the day of the week and the month. Choice *B* is incorrect because it is missing the comma between the day and year. Choice *C* is incorrect because it adds an unnecessary comma between the month and date. Choice *D* is missing the necessary comma between day of the week and the month.

8. D: *Discipline* and *perseverance* are both spelled correctly in choice *d*. These are both considered commonly misspelled words. One or both words are spelled incorrectly in choices A, B, and C.

9. D: In choice D, the word *function* is a noun. While the word *function* can also act as a verb, in this particular sentence it is acting as a noun as the object of the preposition *at*. Choices A and B are incorrect because the word *function* cannot be used as an adjective or adverb.

10. C: Cacti is the correct plural form of the word *cactus*. Choice A (*tomatos*) includes an incorrect spelling of the plural of *tomato*. Both choice B (*analysis*) and choice D (*criterion*) are incorrect because they are in singular form. The correct plural form for these choices would be *criteria* and analyses.

11. B: Quotation marks are used to indicate something someone said. The example sentences feature a direct quotation that requires the use of double quotation marks. Also, the end punctuation, in this case a question mark, should always be contained within the quotation marks. Choice A is incorrect because there is an unnecessary period after the quotation mark. Choice C is incorrect because it uses single quotation marks, which are used for a quote within a quote. Choice D is incorrect because it places the punctuation outside of the quotation marks.

12. D: The prefix *trans* means across, beyond, over. Choices A, B, and C are incorrect because they are the meanings of other prefixes. Choice A is a meaning of the prefix *de*. Choice B is the meaning of the prefix *omni*. Choice C is one of the meanings of the prefix *pro*. The example words are helpful in determining the meaning of *trans*. All of the example words—*transfer, transact, translation, transport*—indicate something being *across, beyond,* or *over* something else. For example, *translation* refers to text going across languages. If no example words were given, you could think of words starting with *trans* and then compare their meanings to try to determine a common definition.

13. D: In choice D, the word *part* functions as an adjective that modifies the word *Irish*. Choices A and C are incorrect because the word *part* functions as a noun in these sentences. Choice B is incorrect because the word *part* functions as a verb.

14. C: *All of Shannon's family and friends* is the complete subject because it includes who or what is doing the action in the sentence as well as the modifiers that go with it. Choice A is incorrect because it only includes the simple subject of the sentence. Choices B and D are incorrect because they only include part of the complete subject.

15. D: Choice D directly addresses the reader, so it is in second person point of view. This is an imperative sentence since it issues a command; imperative sentences have an *understood you* as the subject. Choice A uses first person pronouns *I* and *my*. Choices B and C are incorrect because they use third person point of view.

16. A: The word *prodigious* is defined as very impressive, amazing, or large. In this sentence, the meaning can be drawn from the words *they became nervous about climbing its distant peak*, as this would be an appropriate reaction upon seeing a very large peak that's far in the distance. Choices B, C, and D do not accurately define the word *prodigious*, so they are incorrect.

17. D: Choice D correctly places a hyphen after the prefix *ex* to join it to the word *husband.* Words that begin with the prefixes *great, trans, ex, all,* and *self*, require a hyphen. Choices A and C place hyphens in words where they are not needed. *Beagle mix* would only require a hyphen if coming before the word *Henry*, since it would be serving as a compound adjective in that instance. Choice B contains hyphens that are in the correct place but are formatted incorrectly since they include spaces between the hyphens and the surrounding words.

18. C: Choice *C* is correct because quotation marks should be used for the title of a short work such as a poem. Choices A, B, and D are incorrect because the titles of novels, films, and newspapers should be placed in italics, not quotation marks.

19. A: This question focuses on the correct usage of the commonly confused word pairs of *it's/its* and *then/than*. *It's* is a contraction for *it is* or *it has*. *Its* is a possessive pronoun. The word *than* shows comparison between two things. *Then* is an adverb that conveys time. Choice *C* correctly uses *it's* and *than*. *It's* is a contraction for *it has* in this sentence, and *than* shows comparison between *work* and *rest*. None of the other answers choices use both of the correct words.

20. C: The suffix *-fy* means to make, cause, or cause to have. Choices A, B, and D are incorrect because they show meanings of other suffixes. Choice *A* shows the meaning of the suffix *-ous*. Choice *B* shows the meaning of the suffix *–ist*, and choice D shows the meaning of the suffix *-age*.

21. B: *Dissatisfied* and *accommodations* are both spelled correctly in Choice *B*. These are both considered commonly misspelled words. One or both words are spelled incorrectly in choices A, C, and D.

22. B: Choice *B* is an imperative sentence because it issues a command. In addition, it ends with a period, and an imperative sentence must end in a period or exclamation mark. Choice A is a declarative sentence that states a fact and ends with a period. Choice *C* is an exclamatory sentence that shows strong emotion and ends with an exclamation point. Choice *D* is an interrogative sentence that asks a question and ends with a question mark.

23. A: *After* and *then* are transitional words that indicate time or position. Choice *B* is incorrect because the words *at, with,* and *to* are used as prepositions in this sentence, not transitions. Choice *C* is incorrect because the words *had* and *took* are used as verbs in this sentence. In Choice *D*, *a* and *the* are used as articles in the sentence.

24. C: Choice *C* is a compound sentence because it joins two independent clauses—*The baby was sick* and *I decided to stay home from work*—with a comma and the coordinating conjunction *so*. Choices A, B, and D, are all simple sentences, each containing one independent clause with a complete subject and predicate. Choices A and D each contain a compound subject, or more than one subject, but they are still simple sentences that only contain one independent clause. Choice *B* contains a compound verb (more than one verb), but it's still a simple sentence.

25. A: Choice *A* includes all of the words functioning as nouns in the sentence. Choice *B* is incorrect because it includes the words *final* and *academic,* which are functioning as adjectives in this sentence. The word *he* makes Choice *C* incorrect because it is a pronoun. This example also includes the word *library*, which can function as a noun, but is functioning as an adjective modifying the word *databases* in this sentence. Choice *D* is incorrect because it leaves out the proper noun *Robert*.

26. C: The simple subject of this sentence, the word *lots*, is plural. It agrees with the plural verb form *were*. Choice *A* is incorrect, because the simple subject *there*, referring to the two constellations, is considered plural. It does not agree with the singular verb form *is*. In Choice *B*, the singular subject *four*, does not agree with the plural verb form *needs*. In Choice *D* the plural subject *everyone* does not agree with the singular verb form *have*.

27. B: *Excellent* and *walking* are adjectives modifying the noun *tours*. *Rich* is an adjective modifying the noun *history*, and *brotherly* is an adjective modifying the noun *love*. Choice *A* is incorrect because all of these words are functioning as nouns in the sentence. Choice *C* is incorrect because all of these words are functioning as verbs in the sentence. Choice *D* is incorrect because all of these words are considered prepositions, not adjectives.

28. D: The object pronouns *her* and *me* act as the indirect objects of the sentence. If *me* is in a series of object pronouns, it should always come last in the series. Choice *A* is incorrect because it uses subject pronouns *she* and *I*. Choice *B* is incorrect because it uses the subject pronoun *she*. Choice *C* uses the correct object pronouns, but they are in the wrong order.

29. A: In this example, a colon is correctly used to introduce a series of items. Choice *B* places an unnecessary comma before the word *because*. A comma is not needed before the word *because* when it introduces a dependent clause at the end of a sentence and provides necessary information to understand the sentence. Choice *C* is incorrect because it uses a semi-colon instead of a comma to join a dependent clause and an independent clause. Choice *D* is incorrect because it uses a colon in place of a comma and coordinating conjunction to join two independent clauses.

30. B: Choice *B* correctly uses the contraction for *you are* as the subject of the sentence, and it correctly uses the possessive pronoun *your* to indicate ownership of the jacket. It also correctly uses the adverb *there*, indicating place. Choice *A* is incorrect because it reverses the possessive pronoun *your* and the contraction for *you are*. It also uses the possessive pronoun *their* instead of the adverb *there*. Choice *C* is incorrect because it reverses *your* and *you're* and uses the contraction for *they are* in place of the adverb *there*. Choice *D* incorrectly uses the possessive pronoun *their* instead of the adverb *there*.

31. A: Only two of these suffixes, –*ize* and –*en*, can be used to form verbs, so *B* and *D* are incorrect. Those choices create adjectives. The suffix –*ize* means "to convert or turn into." The suffix –*en* means "to become." Because this sentence is about converting ideas into money, money + –*ize* or *monetize* is the most appropriate word to complete the sentence, so *C* is incorrect.

32. A: Slang refers to non-standard expressions that are not used in elevated speech and writing. Slang tends to be specific to one group or time period and is commonly used within groups of young people during their conversations with each other. Jargon refers to the language used in a specialized field. The vernacular is the native language of a local area, and a dialect is one form of a language in a certain region. Thus, *B*, *C*, and *D* are incorrect.

33. D: Colloquial language is that which is used conversationally or informally, in contrast to professional or academic language. While *ain't* is common in conversational English, it is a non-standard expression in academic writing. For college-bound students, high school should introduce them to the expectations of a college classroom, so *B* is not the best answer. Teachers should also avoid placing moral or social value on certain patterns of speech. Rather than teaching students that their familiar speech patterns are bad, teachers should help students learn when and how to use appropriate forms of expression, so *C* is wrong. *Ain't* is in the dictionary, so *A* is incorrect, both in the reason for counseling and in the factual sense.

34. A: The topic of the passage is Caribbean island destinations. The *topic* of the passage can be described in a one- or two-word phrase. Remember, when paraphrasing a passage, it is important to include the topic. Paraphrasing is when one puts a passage into his or her own words.

35. C: Family or adult-only resorts and activities are supporting details in this passage. *Supporting details* are details that help readers better understand the main idea. They answer questions such as who, what, where, when, why, or how. In this question, cruises and local events are not discussed in the passage, whereas family and adult-only resorts and activities support the main idea.

36. D: Taylor is working on the outlining process. A writer should create an outline after they've come up with the topics and points they want to write about. While this is a type of organization (Choice *A*), it is referred to as "outlining" in the writing process. Drafting (Choice *B*) consists of actually writing the paper, and revising (Choice *C*) occurs after drafting/writing is complete or simultaneously with it.

FREE Test Taking Tips DVD Offer

To help us better serve you, we have developed a Test Taking Tips DVD that we would like to give you for FREE. **This DVD covers world-class test taking tips that you can use to be even more successful when you are taking your test.**

All that we ask is that you email us your feedback about your study guide. Please let us know what you thought about it – whether that is good, bad or indifferent.

To get your **FREE Test Taking Tips DVD**, email freedvd@studyguideteam.com with "FREE DVD" in the subject line and the following information in the body of the email:

a. The title of your study guide.

b. Your product rating on a scale of 1-5, with 5 being the highest rating.

c. Your feedback about the study guide. What did you think of it?

d. Your full name and shipping address to send your free DVD.

If you have any questions or concerns, please don't hesitate to contact us at freedvd@studyguideteam.com.

Thanks again!

Made in the USA
San Bernardino, CA
26 July 2017